How to Protect Your Heart
From Your Doctor

Howard H. Wayne, M.D.
June 1, 1995

How to Protect Your

HEART

From Your Doctor

HOWARD H. WAYNE, M.D., M.S., F.A.C.C

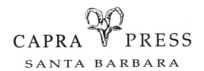

CAPRA PRESS

SANTA BARBARA

*Dedicated to my wife Gypsy, whose love
and support made this book possible,
and to our three children:
Michael, Michelle and Bradley.*

&

Cover design by Frank Goad.
Typography by Jimmy O'Shea.
Author's photo by Gypsy Wayne.

LIBRARY OF CONGRESS CATALOGING-IN-PUBLICATION DATA

Wayne, Howard H.
How to protect your heart from your doctor / Howard H. Wayne.
p. cm.
ISBN 0-88496-383-7
1. Cardiology. 2. Medical errors. I. Title
RC669.W316 1995
616.1'2—dc20   94-15372
                                                        CIP

CAPRA PRESS

Box 2068, Santa Barbara, CA 93120

TABLE OF CONTENTS

Part III: Information to Help Protect Your Heart

FOREWORD:

AN OVERVIEW

THE PAST

SINCE THE BEGINNING OF RECORDED HISTORY, members of the medical profession have occupied a special place in the lives of their fellow men and women. Doctors are given information that is hidden from a best friend, husband or wife. A patient believes what the doctor says with the same complete trust a small child has in his parents. If a special examination, blood test or procedure is advised, the patient readily agrees. If a specimen or sample of one's body is required, it is given. If a test is recommended, even if it carries some risk to health or life, the doctor is allowed to perform whatever is needed. If drugs are said to be necessary, even at the risk of serious side effects, the patient, nonetheless, agrees to their administration. And if the doctor says, "We must operate on you," then permission is granted.

No other profession has held such power over its fellow man for so long . Kings, dictators, presidents, popes, and military commanders have wielded huge power, have ordered men to lay down their lives, and have been obeyed gladly. But such power usually lasts only a moment in time. And while men and women may sacrifice their lives for a cause, how many will risk the lives of their children on the word of a stranger? Yet it is done every day.

Until recently, in principle, as well as in practice, the doctor *was* the medical profession— no other entity was involved. The patient's relationship was only with his doctor. This was the person in whom he placed his trust, and only rarely was it abused. Although doctors of bygone eras could not do much good because of their limited treatment options, neither could they do much harm.

THE PRESENT

ALL THIS HAS CHANGED. As this century draws to a close, the diagnosis and treatment of heart disease is a paradox. At one extreme, millions of Americans with a heart disorder or high blood pressure are unaware of its existence, and are at great risk of suffering a heart attack or dying because overt symptoms have not yet occurred. Yet, we have the technology to diagnose their disease, and treat it before such complications develop. Ironically, in spite of the awesome diagnostic capabilities of that technology, most of it stands uselessly by because our insurance industry, and our health care delivery systems refuse to allow its use in those patients without symptoms. As a consequence, we end up with underdiagnosis and undertreatment of a significant percentage of our population who need medical help.

At the other extreme, patients with symptoms are often overdiagnosed, overtreated, and subjected to unnecessary surgery in incredible numbers. Many may become disabled or die today as the result of complications from needless invasive treatments or surgery. Yet, there exist newer and safer ways of diagnosing and treating heart disease which can transform it from a premature lethal illness, to a relatively benign condition not requiring surgical treatment and compatible with a normal life span.

RESPONSIBILITY FOR HEALTH CARE DECISIONS

DECISIONS FOR MEDICAL CARE were once entirely under the control of a doctor. Now, the responsibility for health care has expanded during the past twenty years to include insurance companies, the federal government, hospitals, and managed health care plans to which both patient and doctor belong.

In addition, a number of other forces exert a powerful effect on health care. These include the employer who pays for the cost of the health plan, the professional organization of which the doctor is a member, the legal system, and even the newspapers and television. Furthermore, how medicine is practiced is enormously influenced by pharmaceutical companies, corporations who manufacture medical equipment, and medical journals that publish scientific articles, many of which are really medical advertisements for some new treatment that is ineffective and occasionally harmful.

Decisions involving what tests to use for making a diagnosis, what diagnosis to give the patient, what drugs are prescribed, and when surgery should be performed can no longer be made solely by the physician. The result has been a gradual transformation of many physicians from dedicated humanitarians concerned about the quality of health care to economically motivated employees of the health care industry. At the same time, health care has become industrialized with profit as the primary objective rather than the welfare of the patient. In the process, the patient often ends up as a casualty, becoming a victim of the medical profession .

EFFECT ON COST

ONE OF THE MOST SIGNIFICANT RESULTS of the change in the way medicine is practiced has been a relentless increase in the cost of medical care. The health care industry has attempted to justify this high cost by claiming that high technology saves lives. This may be true in individual cases. However, the number saved is small and is often offset by lives lost because even ordinary care has become so expensive that it is beyond the reach of many citizens. Thus, benign illnesses that are not treated for lack of money, evolve into deadly afflictions that cripple or kill.

EFFECT ON RESEARCH

NOT ONLY has the practice of medicine changed, but so has research. It has become a highly commercialized big business. Increasingly, untried procedures and treatments are recommended as "the newest form of medical therapy." One of the by-products of such aggressive medical care is the practice of advising a new and controversial form of treatment as if it were the only therapy for a particular medical condition. Typically, the trusting patient is told that the proposed remedy is in widespread use. The inference is that it is preferable. Unfortunately, the patient is not informed as to whether this remedy is actually preferable for him and his condition. Frequently, physicians exaggerate the benefits, and minimize the side effects of these new treatments. As a result, the patient rarely gives truly informed consent. Hospitals and medical centers are all too willing to try these new procedures which the media calls the "latest medical treatment." However, the enthusiasm of the hospitals is not for the advancement of medical knowledge but for the profitability of the treatment.

A system has evolved in which high technology testing and treatment have become a profitable substitute for the once sacred patient-physician relationship. In many instances the patient is no longer an end but a means to an end. He is no longer an individual, but a test subject for the newest diagnostic equipment and treatment purchased by the hospital or medical center. Such treatments are often *not* the latest in medical care but the latest in medical experimentation!

What is worrisome about all of this is that so many of us are at the mercy of so few, and fewer still realize their plight or even understand what is happening. It is essential that the public be made aware of what is happening. It is not always safe to unquestionably accept a doctor's recommended treatment, particularly if it poses some risk to the patient's life.

The medical profession's ancient goal has been to help the sick by preventing and treating illness, and to do so in a manner that is in the best interest of the patient. As you will see in the chapters that follow, this goal is often in conflict with the forces that currently dominate the way medicine is practiced. The outcome, depending upon the type of health plan to which the patient belongs, can be one in which diagnostic tests and treatment are knowingly withheld when they should be given, or, surgery is performed when alternative, less lucrative forms of medical care will work just as well. In the latter case, the treatment may be worse than the disease. In both instances the patient becomes a victim of the doctor, and/or of the health care delivery system of which he is a member.

Yet medicine, nonetheless, remains the noblest of callings. Most doctors are dedicated to saving lives through the appropriate use of modern technology and therapy. It is the misapplication of that technology, the industrialization of health care, and the distortion of the imperative of medicine by outside forces that is destroying the profession. In the process, the doctor is often the innocent tool and the patient a casualty.

Over 200 years ago, the French writer Rousseau said: "Before doctors, people used to die naturally." In his wildest dreams, Rousseau could not possibly have imagined what the practice of medicine would be like near the end of the twentieth century. Yet, what he said long ago is just as true today as it was then. I hope, after reading *How to Protect Your Heart From Your Doctor* you will understand what is happening. Hopefully, this knowledge will allow you to defend yourself against the forces controlling the medical profession and help you avoid unintentional harm, either as a result of underdiagnosis and undertreatment due to inadequate medical care, or overdiagnosis and overtreatment resulting from the desire for high profits.

Part I:

UNDERDIAGNOSIS
and
UNDERTREATMENT

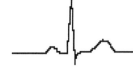

1.

HEART DISEASE

If you have it, your doctor may not be able to detect it.

EACH WEEK IN THE NEXT YEAR, nearly 10,000 Americans will die of a heart attack. One out of five will be less than sixty years old. Another 20,000 will have a heart attack from which they will recover. Nearly two-thirds will have little or no warning of their impending catastrophe, even though more than half will visit a physician only a few months before their tragedy. It is hardly comforting to know that a doctor's examination will fail to alert most of these future victims to their danger. The following case history is just one of the nearly 1,400 disasters that occur each day in the United States alone.

Bill Spenser, an electronics engineer, had just turned 50. As far as he knew he was in reasonably good health. However, he was a cigarette smoker, was moderately overweight, had minimal elevation of his blood pressure, and worked twelve to fourteen hours a day in a stressful job. Accordingly, each year he took the time to have a check-up with his family physician. This year, in particular, Bill had been especially concerned because recently he had begun to experience more fatigue in the evening.

When Bill went in for his examination, he informed the doctor that, except for his tiredness, he felt fine. The doctor checked his weight and blood pressure, listened to his heart with a stethoscope, did a general examination, performed an electrocardiogram (EKG), and drew blood for a blood count and chemistry panel.

Afterwards, Bill was relieved to learn that he had again passed his annual examination. The doctor had remarked that Bill's blood pressure of 145/90 was somewhat higher than before, however, it did not require medication, and probably was related to his stressful job. Since the doctor had found nothing abnormal, Bill assumed his fatigue was job-related.

One night after a particularly stressful day at work, Bill noted a tightness and a fullness in his chest. Though not severe, it was uncomfortable. In addition, he felt somewhat nauseated. He knew it couldn't be his heart because his electrocardiogram just last week had been normal, and the doctor had detected nothing unusual during his examination. Consequently, he felt his distress was due to something he had eaten, and did not become alarmed.

After an hour the discomfort gradually went away. Bill felt somewhat better but very tired, and decided to go to bed early. His wife suggested that he call the doctor in the morning if he didn't feel better. A few hours after going to bed he awoke with the same discomfort. Now it felt like an elephant was sitting on his chest. Again he was nauseated, but this time wanted to throw up. He rose from bed to go to the bathroom, took about five steps and collapsed.

His wife heard a loud crash and jumped out of bed only to see her husband lying in a crumpled heap on the bedroom floor. She tried frantically and unsuccessfully to revive him. Hastily she dialed 911 and asked for the paramedics. When they arrived in fifteen minutes, the victim was blue, pulseless and had dilated, fixed pupils. All attempts at resuscitation failed. Bill was dead.

What had happened? How could Bill receive a clean bill of health the week before, only to die of a massive heart attack? Was this a rare event, or was it common? Had the doctor been negligent or sloppy? Did he make a mistake when he read Bill's electrocardiogram, and was the EKG really normal?

The answers to these questions are not simple. In many instances collapse and death are the initial and only symptoms of coronary disease. Such events can be compared to earthquakes and volcanoes. The outward manifestations are sudden and dramatic; in reality, forces have been at work over a period of years. Collapse, heart attacks, and death are the end result of a silent disease process that progresses for decades.

Heart disease usually remains undetected because the diagnostic procedures available for recognizing these gradual changes are not utilized properly. Thus, we find that many patients who die suddenly, like Bill, have recently been to a doctor and have been told they are in good health.

Had Bill been aware of the limitations of the examination he received, had he known it was not much different than the one given his grandfather two generations ago, he would not have been satisfied with the report received. More importantly, had his checkup been performed with more modern instrumentation, cardiac abnormalities would have been found, and appropriate medication could have been prescribed. Then if Bill and his wife had known that a heart problem existed, they would have called his doctor with the initial onset of his pain, and Bill would have been hospitalized. A heart attack might have been avoided. Had his cardiac arrest occurred in an intensive care unit, he would have received an electric shock to the chest to restart his heartbeat, and his premature death would have been prevented.

Was the doctor guilty of malpractice? Probably not. Malpractice is said to occur when a physician fails to exercise reasonable care in the examination and treatment of a patient, or when the standard of care used is significantly less than what any other family physician would do. What Bill's doctor did was not any different from most doctor's exams. Thus, the error lies not with the doctor, but with the standard of care employed.

To understand why, we must consider the symptoms of heart disease and the medical procedures employed in heart examinations. It would be nice to say that such matters are technical and need only concern doctors. Unfortunately, this is not true. Deplorably, far too many doctors are either unaware of the limitations of their present examination methods or choose to ignore them. Arming yourself with foreknowledge of these limitations could save your life. If you are to avoid the disaster that befell Bill Spenser, it is important that you know what to do should you ever have a similar problem.

SYMPTOMS OF CORONARY ARTERY DISEASE

First you must be aware that most patients with heart disease usually do not have symptoms with ordinary activities until their disease is fairly advanced. When they first sense something is wrong, it may not be signaled by chest pain. In fact, many patients insist that they do not have pain, they experience a tightness, heaviness, or an uncomfortable feeling in their chest. Sometimes the discomfort will radiate to the neck, jaw, left shoulder, or down the inner side of the left arm and forearm. As the individual becomes familiar with the conditions which elicit these feelings, he subconsciously avoids the situations that bring them on. Consequently, when asked if he has any symptoms, the customary answer is "No." If you don't see a doctor until you have severe chest pain or discomfort in your chest upon exertion, it may be too late.

While pain may be the most readily recognized symptom of a heart disorder, it is not the most common indication. Far more frequent is exertional fatigue. If you feel perfectly comfortable at rest, but rapidly tire whenever you do any physical exertion, there is something wrong. Occasionally, your fatigue may be accompanied by shortness of breath. Be careful that you don't attribute your fatigue to aging, or lack of exercise, or overweight. These are very common rationalizations. If your fatigue has come on relatively recently, watch out! There is something wrong, and it must be checked by the appropriate doctor and tests.

Why do many victims of heart disease experience symptoms only when their disease is far advanced? Part of the reason is our modern civilization. Few of us engage in any form of regular exercise or strenuous exertion. In addition, the heart is a wondrously adaptive organ. If an area of heart muscle receives an inadequate amount of blood because of a narrowed coronary artery, its contractions become weaker, or it may be unable to contract at all.

This causes the opposite wall of the heart to compensate by working harder. As a result, the overall function of the heart remains unchanged. Unless the body is subject to extremes of exertion, a decrease in total function is difficult to detect. Consequently, the victim is unaware of any symptoms.

The situation may be likened to two men working to fill a truck with dirt every hour. Then, one becomes ill and is unable to work. As long as the truck pulls out with a full load of dirt every hour, no one suspects anything is wrong. If someone took the time to watch the men, he might find that only one man is doing all the work—at the expense of working twice as hard. As long as only one truckload an hour is all that is needed, the deception will go unnoticed. Suppose, however, the truck has to be filled twice an hour. Now the work requirement has exceeded the ability of one man, and the limitation that results soon becomes apparent. In the same way, the limitations of a patient with heart disease are not apparent with ordinary activities, or even moderate exertion. Not until the physical activity is quite vigorous will chest pain appear.

People who exercise both regularly and strenuously may experience a gradual falling off of performance over a period of a few months to a few years. In spite of their ability to exercise at a high level, they too will notice symptoms but only with very intense activities. Not uncommonly, however, an exercise program may be interrupted because of illness, vacation, or the demands of work. Now, however, attempts at restarting will be met with symptoms at a much lower level of exercise. For any of these signals, an examination by a qualified specialist would be wise.

THE PHYSICAL EXAMINATION FOR HEART DISEASE

You need to know that the common physical examination for heart disease given by most physicians will rarely detect coronary artery disease unless you've had one or more heart attacks. Even then, if the doctor is unaware of such an attack, he may not be able to tell whether the disease is present. How many times have you had such an examination, where the doctor took your blood pressure, listened to your heart with a stethoscope, took an EKG and drew blood for some tests? If you're an older reader, you probably have gone through this same procedure many times—and it's always the same—even if your first examination was forty years ago. That's the kind of examination that Bill Spenser had.

If this examination has been around for so many years, it must be adequate. I know the public believes that, and many doctors do too. The reality is it will detect disease in no more than 10% to 20 % of the patients. The ordinary stethoscope rarely detects the abnormal heart sounds or murmurs that are present in most patients with early or moderate degrees of heart disease. Most doctors can determine whether such sounds or murmurs are absent in less than a minute—they rarely listen longer because there's nothing that can be heard with an ordinary stethoscope.

To understand why, it might do well to compare the heart to an automobile motor. If a motor is not running properly it will often make a noise. One doesn't have to be a mechanic to recognize that something is wrong, since a normally functioning engine is fairly quiet. When the heart is not contracting normally, it also will make noise of several kinds. In medical jargon, the noises are called abnormal heart sounds and heart murmurs. Unfortunately, these abnormal heart sounds have a very low frequency of about 25 Hertz. This frequency is so low it is inaudible to the human ear. If a heart murmur is present, it, too, will be difficult to hear in the early stages of heart disease because these murmurs usually have a very high frequency and are very faint. They are easily masked by the louder, normal heart sounds. Thus, neither the very low frequency, abnormal heart sounds, nor the faint, high frequency heart murmurs that are usually present in patients with early heart disease, can be detected by a standard stethoscope.

THE ELECTROCARDIOGRAM

An EKG measures the electrical conductivity of the heart muscle. This conductivity will not be altered until *after* the muscle is damaged, and that might not be until days or weeks after a heart attack—if you survive. Even when a coronary artery is almost completely closed, as long as blood can get through to nourish the heart muscle, that muscle will remain unharmed and will usually register normal on an EKG taken at rest, although it will not function normally during exercise.

The electrocardiogram does not reflect the performance of the heart. One person might have a clearly abnormal EKG, but be able to run a marathon race. Another individual might have a perfectly normal tracing, but be unable to walk a half a block before chest pain or fatigue appears. The reason for this discordance is that the EKG records only the electrical output of the heart, and not its mechanical function. Consequently, it is no more capable of reflecting the heart's mechanical performance than measuring the voltage in an automobile battery will reflect the performance of the car to which it belongs.

As a result of these limitations, the electrocardiogram is not any more effective than the stethoscope in the early detection of coronary artery disease. It has limited usefulness in those patients who have advanced disease, and in those who have just had a heart attack, but by then it may be too late.

Based upon the principles I have just discussed, it is important for you to be aware that a potential heart victim may have no obvious symptoms and may be able to pass a *routine* physical examination without any abnormalities being discovered. Often, the first symptom of heart disease is death from a heart attack. Even if you have a nonspecific symptom such as exertional fatigue, and a cardiac evaluation shows no abnormal findings, the examining physician may attribute your symptom to another cause such as deconditioning. It is not hard to see why coronary artery disease kills more people than all other diseases combined— it can't be detected!

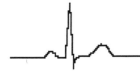

2.

HIGH BLOOD
PRESSURE

*You may have it but your doctor doesn't know it,
or if he knows, he may not know when to treat it.*

E VERY READER OF THIS BOOK has had his blood pressure taken one
or more times. It's simple enough; the cuff slips over the upper arm and is positioned so that when it is inflated it will exert
enough pressure to cause the brachial artery underneath to collapse. A stethoscope is placed over the artery just below the cuff,
and air is allowed to gradually escape. When the pressure inside
the cuff falls below the pressure within the brachial artery, blood
will start to flow. At this point the artery continues to be narrowed because a considerable amount of pressure remains within
the cuff. Consequently, as the blood enters the narrowed artery,
the blood flow becomes turbulent and creates a sound. The pressure at which that sound is created is the systolic pressure. It is
measured by the height, in millimeters, of a column of mercury
that can be supported by the pressure within the cuff. This represents the pressure within the heart's left ventricle when the heart
is contracting. Each time the left ventricle contracts, more blood
enters the artery to create another sound. When the pressure
within the cuff falls below the pressure within the artery, it returns to its normal diameter. Accordingly, the blood flow is no

longer turbulent, and there are no more sounds. The pressure at which this occurs is called the diastolic pressure. It represents the pressure within the circulatory system while the heart is relaxing.

Traditionally, one is supposed to be quiet and relaxed when blood pressure is taken. Indeed, if the blood pressure is found to be elevated, many physicians will have the patient relax in a quiet room and recheck the pressure ten to fifteen minutes later. As a result, patients may live with an elevated blood pressure for years before it is finally detected. High blood pressure is to the development of coronary artery disease and heart attacks what high speed is to the occurrence of automobile accidents. Failure to identify high blood pressure in a patient with early heart disease, may be equivalent to signing his death warrant.

Normal blood pressure varies between 100 to 135 millimeters for the systolic pressure, and 60 to 85 millimeters for the diastolic pressure. Pressures above these levels should be considered elevated. The medical term for high blood pressure is hypertension. It wasn't too long ago that hypertension wasn't considered present unless the blood pressure went as high as 160/105. Indeed, it was generally believed that blood pressure was supposed to rise as we aged. We now know that this is not true—if pressure increases with age, you have hypertension.

FREQUENCY OF HYPERTENSION

The National Heart and Lung Institute tells us that a quarter of our population have or will develop hypertension. Perhaps 50% to 60% of them are aware that their pressure has been elevated on at least one occasion. Probably no more than 10% to 20% of these are receiving an adequate amount of medication. Failure to detect hypertension can be disastrous, as we can see in the following story.

Frank Holt was a 50-year-old human resources director of a biomedical firm. For the past few months he had been experiencing chest pain. Under stress he felt a tightness across his whole chest. Disciplining an employee or giving a report at a meeting was particularly stressful. On one occasion he had to excuse himself from a meeting. It was nearly an hour before the discomfort in his chest subsided. Even at night, when he was trying to go to sleep, he could feel his heart pounding. In addition, he noticed that when he played tennis or climbed stairs, the old stamina was simply not there. At the end of the work day he often felt exhausted. His company had a health plan with one of the medical clinics in his city so he arranged for a complete examination.

Frank went for his examination. He told the doctors of the discomfort in his chest. They took his weight, his resting blood pressure and studied him from top to bottom. They took an electrocardiogram, a chest x-ray, blood tests, urine, stool; they even studied the lower end of his colon with a long instrument known as a sigmoidoscope. Then they placed an array of electrodes on his chest, attached the wires to a small microcomputer that clipped to his belt, and recorded, and analyzed every single heart beat over the next twenty-four hours—all 115,000 of them. Then Frank had a treadmill test. All the doctors could find with these tests was a blood pressure they felt was on the borderline of being elevated. They did not think this was significant.

Frank was informed that in spite of the fact his tests were normal, there was still a possibility he had coronary artery disease. Frank was asked to undergo a coronary angiogram. He entered the hospital the following week, and the angiogram was performed without incidence. One of his coronary arteries was about 70% narrowed and he was told it was responsible for his chest discomfort.

Since he was already on the catheterization table and in position, the cardiologist recommended he have an angioplasty. It was explained to him that this would increase the blood flow through the artery, and eliminate the cause of his chest pain. Frank consented to the procedure, and it was carried out successfully. He was sent home and allowed to return to work within a few days. He was not given any medication. The bill amounted to nearly $12,000. Fortunately his insurance covered most of the expense. He felt lucky he hadn't had bypass surgery and that he didn't have to take any pills.

Six weeks later Frank again began to experience chest pain and pounding of his heart. His illness had resulted in him falling behind in his work; consequently, he was under more stress than ever. Reluctantly, he called the cardiologist who had done his angiogram. He was reassured that up to 40% of patients who undergo angioplasty had a return of their symptoms. All that was necessary was to put another balloon in the artery and dilate it a little bit more vigorously!

Frank reentered the hospital. Once again his blood pressure was found to be borderline elevated on admission, but it became perfectly normal by the next morning. Consequently, it was ignored. His angioplasty was repeated with the balloon inflated to ten atmospheres of pressure (150 lb. per square inch). The balloon was allowed to remain inflated much longer than before. This time, however, a problem developed. While the balloon was inflated, Frank's heart began to beat irregularly, and then went into ventricular fibrillation. Instead of his heart contracting forcefully about once a second, the muscle developed tiny ripples of movement, not unlike the tiny waves one sees when a rock is dropped into a pond. Had this happened anywhere other than on an operating room table or in the intensive care unit of a hospital, he would have died. In this modern age, the cardiologist put paddle electrodes over his heart, and administered an electrical charge. Within moments his heart was beating normally.

Two days later Frank was told he would be fine and was allowed to return home. Still no medication was required. All went well for two months when once more he began to experience chest pains. Again he called the cardiologist. This time he was told that since angioplasty had failed, he would have to have coronary artery bypass surgery. Frank dutifully returned to the hospital making no attempt to seek another opinion.

Frank had his bypass surgery, fortunately without any serious complications. The bill was considerably higher on this occasion—$40,000. Also, this time he had to take off a full two months from work. He was finally pain free—but for only six months. Again his symptoms returned.

Finally Frank decided to see someone else. This time he vowed to find a cardiologist that was not so surgically oriented. That proved to be a problem but finally he located such an individual and made an appointment. This cardiologist carried out a few tests that the medical clinic had omitted. The first abnormality detected was the level to which his blood pressure rose under stress. At rest it was mildly elevated at 150/100. However, when the doctor measured his pressure while Frank squeezed a device known as a hand grip dynamometer, it rose to 225/135 within 60 seconds. Next, the cardiologist listened to his heart with special audiovisual equipment designed to detect abnormal low frequency heart sounds that are usually inaudible with an ordinary stethoscope. Typically such sounds are present only in individuals whose blood pressure is elevated most of the day. Frank had such sounds. This was followed by imaging the pattern of filling and emptying of Frank's heart with a test known as an apexcardiogram. Finally, an echocardiogram was performed. This is a test in which the cardiologist is able to look inside of the heart with a sonar-like device and visualize the heart's chambers.

It was apparent to the new cardiologist that the patient's heart was enlarged and the muscle thickened. All walls were contracting very dynamically. The cardiologist had seen these findings many times before. They were quite typical of hypertension. Frank's symptoms were never due to his coincidental and mild coronary artery disease; they were due to his elevated blood pressure!

The cardiologist explained to Frank that when his blood pressure was elevated during periods of stress, the increased pressure was transmitted to the inside of the heart where it exerted pressure against the heart muscle. The increase in pressure within the heart muscle itself compressed the small blood vessels throughout the muscle causing a reduction in blood flow. This caused chest pain just as effectively as the narrowing of a coronary artery. The cardiologist called this hypertensive angina.

Not only did Frank have pain from a reduction in blood flow, but his heart contracted much more vigorously under stress. As a result, his heartbeat was more forceful—forceful enough so that it was hitting against his chest from the inside of the chest cavity. A few strong beats against his chest from the inside would not be felt. However, if Frank were under stress for a couple of hours it would add up to 5,000 to 10,000 beats. That could give anybody chest pain.

The cardiologist put Frank on blood pressure medicine. In six weeks Frank's blood pressure was 115/70, he felt better, his chest pains and pounding were completely gone, and he began to experience a return of his old vigor. Gradually his exercise tolerance returned as his deconditioning from all his inactivity disappeared. Why didn't the doctors at the medical clinic treat his elevated blood pressure first? Then, if his symptoms had failed to disappear, they could have proceeded with the angiograms, angioplasty and bypass surgery. Frank asked the new cardiologist about that, but the doctor was too polite to respond.

SIGNS AND SYMPTOMS OF HYPERTENSION

In order to understand why so many people with hypertension have neither been diagnosed nor treated, a certain amount of background information is necessary. Most doctors still believe patients with high blood pressure do not have symptoms, and the diagnosis can be made only if the blood pressure is elevated. Accordingly, if the pressure is normal or near normal upon examination, then the disease is not considered to be present. Implicit in this concept is the conviction that our blood pressure is approximately as stable as our weight. In other words, if the patient's pressure in the doctor's office was 120/80, then it will be 120/80 almost all the time. None of these assumptions is true.

Clinical experience has shown that most individuals with early hypertension have symptoms, particularly when they work under stress. For example, a victim will often note more forceful beating of his heart, irregular heart beats, excessive or inappropriate sweating, headaches, and a feeling of tenseness or nervousness. Exercise often brings a noticeable loss of stamina and a pounding of the heart. In addition, a hypertensive patient will demonstrate certain abnormalities during a medical evaluation besides his increased blood pressure. Typically he will have a florid or reddish coloration of his face. When one feels the heart of such a patient, the forceful beating can be easily discerned. Moreover, sounds generated by that heart are much louder than sounds coming from a normal heart. Even the pulse seems stronger. Finally, an echocardiogram or ultrasound evaluation will show enlargement of the heart's chambers and increased thickness of its muscle. It is interesting to note however, that the EKG is always normal at this stage of the disease.

All these abnormalities may exist in many people who have the same complaints as the hypertensive patient, yet their blood pressure is normal at rest. They have a form of hidden hypertension. If such a patient has his pressure taken while undergoing a mild stress, such as maximally squeezing a rubber ball, a remarkable and precipitous increase in blood pressure almost invariably occurs. The systolic pressure may rise by 70 to 90 millimeters and the diastolic pressure by 30 to 45 millimeters. Thus, if the patient's blood pressure is 135/85 in the absence of stress, it may increase to 220/130 in less than 60 seconds! In contrast, a normal individual who has no symptoms, and exhibits none of the abnormalities seen in the hidden hypertensive patient, will show a rise in both the systolic and diastolic blood pressure of no more than 10 to 15 millimeters of mercury.

Over the years I have seen these two distinct responses, one normal and the other abnormal, in many hundreds of patients. The ones with acute elevation of their blood pressure during stress almost invariably have either an elevated blood pressure at rest, or a borderline "normal pressure" such as 135-140/85-90. Many of those with a so-called normal pressure exhibit one or more symptoms or signs of hidden hypertension. Conversely, those patients who show a minimal increase in pressure with stress, do not have any of the symptoms of hypertension, nor any of the abnormal findings noted on examination or testing.

BLOOD PRESSURE CONTROL MECHANISM

From these observations we can conclude that some form of feedback control prevents a rise in blood pressure in the normal person when he is stressed. This should not be surprising since many feedback control mechanisms exist in the body. Body temperature is one such system. Regardless of whether it is cold or hot, our body temperature hovers around 98.6 degrees. If it is cold, we shiver to generate internal heat. If it is hot, we perspire to cool the body down. Other feedback control systems exist—if our blood sugar falls below a certain level we feel hungry, if we need water we become thirsty.

It is safe to assume that a blood pressure control system exists in every normal person. When blood pressure starts to rise, the body attempts to lower it by stimulating the blood vessels throughout the body to dilate or enlarge. This probably accounts for the florid or reddish coloration of the face of the hypertensive patient. In contrast, if blood pressure falls abruptly, blood vessels throughout the body constrict, and resistance in the circulatory system increases as the body attempts to bring the blood pressure up. This is why someone who is about to faint gets "as white as a sheet."

NEW DEFINITION OF HYPERTENSION

We now see that hypertension is a malfunction of the blood pressure regulatory mechanism. Such a malfunction may take many years to develop. This means that the feedback control apparatus in these victims operates imperfectly. In the early years of hypertension development, an individual with an imperfect feedback control mechanism may do quite well when not under any tension, and have a normal pressure. However, as soon as tension occurs, the blood pressure quickly rises. The greater the stress, and the longer it exists, the higher the blood pressure, and the longer it remains elevated. Once the stress is gone, the blood pressure gradually returns to normal levels.

As the years go by, the blood pressure regulatory mechanism becomes even less effective, and the victim's blood pressure response becomes worse, with peaks and valleys throughout the day, depending upon the level of strain. By this time, periods of tension are accompanied or followed by symptoms, and the patient may see a physician. As a rule, since he is away from his tension provoking environment, his blood pressure will be found to be normal or borderline, and a routine examination will fail to uncover any abnormalities, unless the doctor knows how to look for hidden hypertension. Typically the patient is told there is nothing wrong or he is given a tranquilizer for his "nerves."

In time, the blood pressure peaks and valleys become more frequent, and the valleys do not quite return to normal levels. Eventually, even the valleys are elevated. By this time, the victim's hypertension has become more advanced, and it is now easier to diagnose. This doesn't mean it will be treated unless he has developed one or more complications of his disease.

Even when the blood pressure is mildly elevated, many doctors will not treat such patients. These physicians still hold to the mistaken belief that a blood pressure of 140-150/90-95 is within normal limits, whereas any pressure much above 135-140/85 is too high. This erroneous notion has probably been responsible for more errors in diagnosis, and more unnecessary heart attacks and strokes than all other cardiac risk factors combined!

WHY DOCTORS ARE RELUCTANT TO TREAT MILD HYPERTENSION

Doctors are often reluctant to put patients with mildly elevated pressures on medication because of their concern about the side effects of drugs, the cost, and the usual need to take such medication for life. They ignore the fact that the side effects of a drug are rarely serious, and can be avoided by lowering the dosage. These physicians fail to acknowledge that the side effects of *not* taking medication may be disastrous, and can be far more costly than the price of the medication. Sooner or later, mild hypertension becomes more severe. Many victims with borderline pressures continue for years without appropriate treatment until some major complication finally occurs. Even if a heart attack or stroke does not materialize, we now have evidence that elevated blood pressure causes premature aging of the heart. Furthermore, in those people with coexisting coronary artery disease, chest pain or discomfort may lead to unnecessary angiograms or bypass surgery.

WHAT YOU CAN DO TO FIND OUT
IF YOUR BLOOD PRESSURE IS ELEVATED

What can you do to determine whether you might have unsus-pected hypertension, or have a high risk of getting it? First, pur-chase a self-taking blood pressure cuff. This is a blood pressure device with the listening end of a stethoscope attached to the cuff. It is designed so that the diaphragm of the stethoscope can be placed on the upper arm directly over the brachial artery. The cuff is made so that it can be applied with one hand. The ear pieces of the stethoscope are inserted in the ears and the cuff is inflated. Full directions for doing this accompany the apparatus. As a rule, electronic blood pressure cuffs with digital readouts are not as reliable as the non-electronic variety. Although listen-ing for the sounds over the artery is not as convenient as a digital display, the increased accuracy is worth your effort.

Once you learn how, take your pressure at different times dur-ing the day. It will usually register higher during the morning hours. Find your peak highs and lows. Don't take your pressure just when it is convenient, or when you have the time. These might be stress free periods. Take it when it is inconvenient and you are rushing to get someplace. It is more likely to be elevated then.

Certain groups are prone to high blood pressure. For example, if you have a parent or sibling with hypertension, the odds are very high that you will as well. Stress is another major factor that predisposes you to an elevated blood pressure. If you have a stress-ful job, check your blood pressure frequently at work, particu-larly during periods of tension. Obviously, this is not always convenient, but it is relatively easy to take your blood pressure in the nearest rest room. Typically the blood pressure will be mildly elevated in those who are destined to develop hypertension. At night, however, in the relaxed atmosphere of your home, your pressure probably will be normal.

Be on guard if you find that you like to have a drink at regular intervals when you get home. Early hypertension is often accompanied by nervousness, tenseness, irritability, headaches, and inappropriate sweating. As one of the oldest of tranquilizers, alcohol is often used to relieve these symptoms. Similarly, if you find that you are more short-tempered, or you now have frequent arguments with your spouse, check your blood pressure afterwards. You might be surprised. I have saved many marriages by placing patients with unsuspected hypertension on blood pressure medication.

If you find your blood pressure is elevated during stress, but normal at rest, you still do not have conclusive proof you have hypertension. The next step is to prove that your blood pressure is elevated during most of the day. This is not easy to do. Fortunately, there are two kinds of tests that will shed some light upon the problem. The most important is the echocardiogram. This test will allow the doctor to determine if your heart chambers are enlarged and the muscle is thickened. These changes invariably occur only if your pressure is elevated most of the day. The second test that can be employed is a stress test. Normally during a stress test, the systolic pressure rises, and the diastolic pressure falls because of the immense amounts of blood required by the exercising muscle. Individuals with hypertension behave differently. Both the systolic and diastolic pressure rise. Long term studies have shown that when this happens the subject will usually develop sustained hypertension within the next few years.

With these facts in mind, if your blood pressure levels are elevated, you will need to find a physician willing to treat you medically. Take your records to your doctor and tell him if any of your family members have hypertension. Ask for an echocardiogram and a stress test. If he declines, persist until you find a doctor willing to work with you.

HOW TO DETERMINE IF YOUR BLOOD PRESSURE IS BEING ADEQUATELY TREATED

Once you have started on blood pressure medication, how can you determine if your pressure is under proper control? If you originally had symptoms with your hypertension, then those symptoms will disappear. However, a patient often will not recognize the fact that symptoms were present until after his pressure is under control and he starts to feel well again. On specific questioning he will usually admit he is less nervous, has more energy, the stress he thought was present is gone, and he is sleeping better. He also is less irritable. I recall one patient who said his only complaint since being on medication was that his employees could no longer tell when he was mad because he no longer developed a red face!

There are other ways to determine if blood pressure control is adequate. You could, of course, continue to take your own blood pressure at regular intervals. If your medication is effective, the readings will be significantly lower. A relatively new procedure, not yet widely available, is called ambulatory blood pressure recordings. With this technique, the subject wears a blood pressure cuff for 24 hours. Blood pressure is taken at intervals throughout the day, and the information is recorded on a microchip. Thus, if the blood pressure becomes elevated only during stress, that information will be quickly apparent. At the moment, ambulatory blood pressure recordings are considered by insurance companies to be in the realm of research, and, therefore, are not reimbursable. This is one more example of how the insurance industry attempts to control the practice of medicine.

There are still other ways to determine if medication is effective in controlling your blood pressure. If a repeat stress test is performed while you are on medication, the increase in pressure during exercise will be much lower. Although your diastolic pressure still may not go down, it should no longer rise. And finally, a repeat echocardiogram a year or two after medication is started will typically show a decrease in the size of your heart, assuming it was increased when you started.

Although effective treatment of hypertension can be readily accomplished with just a few of the many drugs that are available, I often see patients who continue to have symptoms. They have been to another doctor, one who treats them with only one drug. Their blood pressure still rises precipitously during stress, although it may be normal at rest. Almost invariably these victims are not being treated with a diuretic and are at risk of major complications. Doctors who attempt to treat hypertension without diuretics have often been mislead into thinking diuretics are harmful by pharmaceutical companies trying to sell their own blood pressure lowering drugs. They are told that diuretics elevate cholesterol and blood sugar levels, and that patients treated with diuretics are at increased risk of having a heart attack. Such claims are ludicrous and have never been documented. Indeed, patients are in greater danger of a heart attack when they are not on a diuretic. Although the cholesterol and blood sugar levels do show a mild increase on diuretic therapy, such an increase is always transient and the levels adjust within a few months. This will be discussed more fully in later chapters. Suffice to say here that often it is difficult to bring a patient's blood pressure to optimal levels without a diuretic. It is to be emphasized that diuretics are perfectly safe, and that the official recommendation of the Joint Commission on Hypertension is that diuretics should be *initially* used in the treatment of high blood pressure.

Remember, hypertension is a lethal disease and frequently exists without symptoms. Even when symptoms are present, they are often attributed to stress. If the symptom is chest pain (hypertensive angina), a common mistake is to assume the pain is due to coronary artery disease and often the patient has to undergo unnecessary angiograms, angioplasty or bypass surgery. A diagnosis of hypertension may not be made until it has been present for many years, and already has produced a complication such as an enlarged heart or a heart attack at a young age. Even then, the blood pressure may be normal at rest, but elevated only during stress. The echocardiogram is the best test to determine if the heart has become enlarged from the increased pressure. The EKG will not show changes unless severe hypertension has been present for many years. Both an echocardiogram and a stress test are mandatory if an elevated blood pressure is suspected. The treatment of hypertension is relatively easy but almost always requires the use of a diuretic.

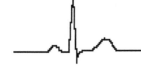

3.

STRESS

A major cause of premature heart disease,
or, my doctor gave me a tranquilizer instead
of heart medicine.

STRESS AS A CAUSE OF HEART DISEASE and high blood pressure has been down played by the medical profession for many years. There are a number of reasons for this reticence. Stress cannot be measured, nor can a number be placed on the response of an individual to stress. A given stress in one person may not even be perceived as such in another. Furthermore, when stress is present all the time, it becomes the norm and is no longer recognized as such. Consequently, most doctors fail to take stress into consideration in diagnosing and treating patients with heart disease.

Can damage occur to a heart repeatedly subjected to strain and tension? Is there a difference between the effects of physical and emotional stress? Physical strain may result in enlargement of the heart and thickening of its muscle in much the same way that lifting weights cause a weight lifter's muscles to enlarge. This would not create any damage or destruction except in extreme instances. Emotional stress is another story as the following case history illustrates.

George Thompson was an upwardly mobile, 47-year old executive. Intensely driven, he had risen in his job from a mechanical engineer in a space program subcontracting firm to president of the company. He was constantly pushing himself, as well as his subordinates, to greater production goals in less and less time. In his eagerness to get defense contracts he would overcommit his manufacturing plant. Often he would find himself in the position of not having the trained personnel, or even the raw material to do the job properly. Overtime, harassment, impatience, cost overruns and rejected parts by the prime contractor had become almost routine. He began to become impatient, short tempered, irritable, tense and unable to sleep. Family problems surfaced frequently; there was rarely time to go out with his wife, except those instances when he brought along a prospective customer. Even then he would spend the whole evening talking business. The children hardly knew what their father looked like. Not surprisingly, discipline problems were frequent. Sixteen hour days were the rule. Traveling became a way of life as his company constantly required him to visit different suppliers and customers.

To relax, George began drinking—just one or two cocktails in the evening. It wasn't very long before this increased; a few martinis during lunch with a client, a couple before heading for home, and three or four more during the evening to help him go to sleep. Soon his weight rose; when his clothes became too tight, that was no problem because he made a lot of money and could buy new ones.

Then the headaches began. After that, he noticed heart palpitations. At first George took aspirin for the pain and experienced only partial relief. Next he used some of his wife's codeine, but that failed as well. Finally he decided to seek professional help. The doctor was busy the day of his visit; George had to wait for some time. He really didn't mind; there were some good magazines in the waiting room; besides, the doctor was a personal friend. When finally examined, he was comparatively relaxed.

George told the doctor about the headaches, his trouble sleeping, and the tenseness, but added that he was under a considerable amount of strain at work. The doctor took his blood pressure, examined his heart with a standard stethoscope, took an electrocardiogram and drew blood for some tests. He was told finally that there was nothing really wrong; the headaches were tension headaches and his blood pressure was just borderline 150/90; he didn't need blood pressure medication. According to the doctor, drugs used to treat high blood pressure had side effects; his pressure wasn't high enough to start such medication. George received a prescription for tranquilizers and reassurance that his symptoms were due to his nerves.

The tranquilizers did help him relax and, when used with aspirin, gave him relief from the headaches. He continued his old ways at the plant working fourteen to sixteen or more hours a day. One evening, while dining with a business client, he began to feel funny. There was a terrible crushing pain in his chest. He began to feel nauseated, rose to go to the restroom, and collapsed. Luck was with George, a doctor dining in the same restaurant administered cardiac resuscitation measures—George's heart had stopped! He was taken to the intensive care unit of the nearest hospital. Tests revealed he had sustained a massive heart attack. The whole front portion of his heart had been destroyed!

George spent the next four months recovering. When he finally was able to return to work, he would tire easily. He simply did not have the stamina to put in more than a few hours a day. A walk across the plant brought on shortness of breath, and sometimes chest pain. He could no longer handle his job. In due time George was asked to step down; shortly thereafter, his job was terminated.

George was shocked, depressed, and angry. He had spent so much time and energy for his company, had suffered a major heart attack, and had been dumped without even as much as a "thank you" from the company owners. He decided to consult an attorney to see if he could claim his heart attack had been the result of stress. His attorney referred him to a physician who specialized in disability work. He received a cursory examination, his hospital record was reviewed and he was politely told there was insufficient evidence that stress would cause heart attacks. Besides, wasn't he having dinner at the time the heart attack started? Eating dinner certainly could not be considered stressful. George did not have a case. To make matters worse, since his termination he has had difficulty obtaining any kind of a job because of his heart attack.

The story I have just described is true; only names and minor details have been changed in order to avoid identification. Is there a relation between stress and heart disease? Does it have any influence on the development of high blood pressure? Can a heart attack be caused by stress? If George's regular doctor had treated his patient properly, would the outcome have been any different?

HISTORICAL OBSERVATIONS ON STRESS

Sudden death due to emotional stress has been described since the existence of written records, even in the Bible. In ancient Rome, the Emperor Nerva was said to have died of a "violent excess of anger" when he was insulted by a senator. Chilean of Lacadaemon is reported to have succumbed from joy while embracing his son who had won the prize at the Olympic games. Pope Innocent IV died suddenly from the "morbid effects of grief" following the calamitous defeat of his army by Manfred. King Philip V of Spain dropped dead when he was informed his army had been defeated.

In 1628 Sir William Harvey, the English scientist who was the first to describe the circulation of blood, declared, "A mental disturbance provoking pain, excessive joy, hope or anxiety extends to the heart, where it affects its temper and rate, impairing general nutrition. It is no wonder many serious diseases thus gain access to the body, when it is suffering from faulty nourishment and lack of normal warmth." Clearly, Harvey's observations were centuries ahead of his time.

STUDIES FROM THE EARLY 20TH CENTURY

In the first half of this century only sporadic attention was directed to the relationship between emotional stress and heart disease. In 1920 the eminent physician Sir William Osler noted, "In a group of 20 men with angina pectoris, [chest pain due to heart disease] every one of whom I knew personally, the outstanding feature was the incessant treadmill of practice; and yet, if hard work alone was responsible, would there not be a great many more cases? Every one of these men had an added factor—worry; in not one single case under 50 years of age was this feature absent."

Because of the inherent difficulties of collecting and documenting data in cases of sudden death, the acquisition of such information and its relation to emotional stress has been difficult. Since such events are totally unexpected, and associated with shock and grief to the family and friends, it would be impractical, if not impossible, to carry out any kind of formal study. Consequently, no further work was carried out until the middle of this century when Dr. George Engel, of the University of Rochester School of Medicine, approached the problem in a novel way. With the aid of friends and colleagues throughout the country, and over a period of years, he collected from newspaper reports, 170 examples of emotional stress resulting in sudden death. Apparently, there seemed to be a relationship.

MODERN STUDIES ON STRESS

In 1958, Dr. Howard Rusk from New York City studied the hereditary background, diet, mode of life, and sources of tension in 100 patients between the ages of twenty-five and forty who had known coronary artery disease. His observations were compared to a similar control group of 100 normal subjects. Heredity was a factor in 67% of the coronary patients compared to 40% of the controls. Fifty percent of the coronary patients ate excessive amounts of fat in their diet compared to 20% of the controls. However, emotional stress associated with job responsibility appeared to be far more significant than either diet or heredity; severe emotional strain was found in 91% of the coronary patients but in only 20% of the normal controls.

In 1965 Dr. Rusk studied 12,000 professional men in fourteen different occupations. He found a marked increase in coronary heart disease with increasingly stressful work. This was particularly evident in individuals between forty and forty-nine years old where the frequency of heart disease was 6 times that of those with low stress jobs.

EFFECTS OF STRESS IN ANIMALS

At about the same time these observations were taking place, the phenomena of stress began to be studied in animals, particularly in pigs. For hundreds of years it had been recognized that the organs of this animal resembled those of humans. For example, a twelfth century anatomy text from Salerno stated, "Although some animals, such as monkeys, are found to resemble ourselves in external form, there are none so like us internally as the pig." Interest in stress initially developed in the late sixties when increasing numbers of unexpected deaths developed among market-sized pigs. During routine handling and moving, red and white areas of discoloration of the skin were noted in the pigs, along with an increase in body temperature. If the stress were continued, the animal developed signs of heart failure and died in an acute shock like state. This phenomena was termed the porcine stress syndrome (PSS). Death often could be prevented by treatment with sedatives, indicating an important factor was stress.

In subsequent studies, when stress was produced in pigs by immobilization, every animal developed significant changes in its electrocardiogram, and some died. All animals, whether they survived or not, showed a unique type of damage to the heart muscle. Such damage, however, was only visible under a microscope. In other words, merely looking at the heart in the PSS cases was not sufficient to detect damage. Of considerable interest was the simultaneous observation that following periods of stress sufficient to produce damage to the heart, an adrenalin like substance, known as catecholamines, could be found in the pig's blood.

RELATIONSHIP BETWEEN STRESS AND ADRENALIN

Fortunately, at this time, the drug Inderal became available for general use. It was, and still is, one of the most important medications for the treatment of coronary artery disease. It belongs to a class of compounds known as beta blockers. These drugs block the effects of adrenaline-like substances upon the heart. These hormones are capable of speeding up the heart rate, elevating blood pressure, increasing energy release from available body glucose and accelerating the clotting of blood. These are all relics of our caveman days when we had to fight for survival or flee. Each represents one of the ways the body prepares us for a life threatening situation. For example, if we are injured our blood will clot faster and prevent us from bleeding to death. Exercise, anger, fright and other emotions will normally increase our heart rate to a considerable degree. Under the influence of Inderal, the heart rate will barely rise, or will stay the same. Predictably, when pigs were pre-treated with Inderal before they were restrained, they did not die or show damage to their hearts. These findings clearly incriminate stress as the cause of their cardiac damage and death.

The finding of increased blood levels of an adrenaline-like substance in stressed animals stimulated further investigations. Attempts were made to find out whether these naturally produced catecholamines could damage the heart when injected into dogs and rats. When these animals were sacrificed and autopsied, massive areas of tissue destruction were found in their hearts similar to that seen after an obstruction of a coronary artery. Animals studied several months later were found to have enlarged hearts and localized areas of weakening known as aneurysms. All had persistent changes in their electrocardiograms. An interesting finding was that many of these animals had normal coronary arteries.

STRESS IN PRIMATES

Of course it was only a matter of time before experiments were begun on primates. An interesting but rather gruesome series of studies was performed on monkeys. Animals were studied in pairs with both monkeys receiving electric shocks at regular intervals. One monkey of a pair was taught how to avoid some of the shocks; it was called the avoidance monkey. Although both groups received the same number of shocks, most of the non-avoidance monkeys showed physical deterioration, marked slowing of the heart, a variety of electrocardiographic changes and ultimately, cardiac arrest. In contrast, most of the avoidance monkeys survived. At autopsy, the avoidance monkeys had normal heart muscle while the non-avoidance animals exhibited areas of destruction. Obviously, it was not the shocks which were so stressful, but the inability to do anything about it.

Other primate studies by Russian investigators have used baboons. The scientists separated dominant, male baboons from their mates and offspring. In full view of the separated male, another male was introduced into the female's cage. The particular species of baboons selected for study developed strong family attachments; consequently, the displaced male showed intense agitation. After several months, high blood pressure and other evidence of cardiovascular disease developed, including electrocardiographic evidence of coronary artery disease. Six of the father baboons had an acute heart attack.

While not part of a formal study on stress, the well known animal observer, Jane Goodall, followed the activities of a tribe of chimpanzees for many years. One particular young chimp was abnormally dependent upon its mother, long beyond the time it should have been completely independent. Although perfectly capable of feeding and defending itself, it seemed to cling to its mother wherever she went. When the mother died accidentally, the young chimp showed all the signs of profound grief. Within a few weeks it, too, died. Had an autopsy been performed, I have no doubt that extensive damage to the heart would have been seen.

Another investigation studied two groups of monkeys maintained on a diet low in fat and containing almost no cholesterol. One group was subjected to high stress induced by such conditions as crowding, the introduction of strangers in the group, and competition for females. After a suitable period of time, the animals were sacrificed and autopsied. Extensive arteriosclerosis of the coronary arteries was seen in the stress group of monkeys but not in the non-stressed, control animals. These findings indicated that even in the absence of fat and cholesterol in the diet, stress alone may cause severe hardening of the arteries.

STUDIES IN HUMANS

When these animal studies were done, the medical profession was preoccupied with the cholesterol theory of heart attacks. Most doctors gave little credence to any relationship between emotional stress and heart disease. Therefore, these animal experiments were important because they helped to renew the interest in this area. In the seventies, several formal investigations uncovered a relationship between long-standing stress in individuals who developed heart attacks, especially if the stress occurred shortly before the attack. Many of these patients expressed a dissatisfaction with their achievements and had a pre-existing depression. This enabled one group of researchers to predict the likelihood of sudden death among those who had suffered a heart attack two months or more in the past.

DEATH FROM STRESS

An interesting set of studies was done on victims of assaults who were hurt but survived without internal injuries. The majority showed microscopic changes in their hearts similar to those described in animals dying of stress. In several instances the victims died even though they hadn't been physically injured. In these cases severe coronary artery disease was found at autopsy. The interesting question was raised as to whether these crimes should be considered homicide as a result of the attack.

If stress is responsible for premature deaths in individuals with unsuspected heart disease, then there should be an increase in people dying during times of natural disasters. This proved to be the case following the Athens earthquake of 1981. An excess of deaths from cardiac causes was found for several days following the quake, but no excess of deaths from other causes. The investigators doing the study felt the responsible mechanism was psychological stress working on a background of underlying cardiac disease.

Interest next developed about the mechanisms of premature deaths. Led by Dr. Bernard Lown of Harvard, attention focused upon the irregular rhythm of the heart in many patients with more advanced forms of heart disease. In 1976, Dr. Lown and his associates had the opportunity to study numerous irregular heart beats and two episodes of cardiac arrest in a thirty-nine year old male patient with normal coronary arteries and serious psychiatric problems. Subsequently, 19 additional patients with advanced degrees of irregular cardiac rhythms were investigated. When they were deliberately exposed to psychological stress, the majority developed a significant increase in the irregularity of their heart rhythm.

Other studies looked at patients when they were driving or speaking publicly. The investigators found not only irregular cardiac rhythms, but changes characteristic of inadequate amounts of blood flow to the heart muscle during those times of stress.

JOB STRESS, HEART ATTACKS
AND PREMATURE DEATHS

A variety of studies looked at the relationships between job stress, heart attacks and premature deaths. A hectic and psychologically demanding job increases the risk of both. Two studies in Norway and Sweden attempted to evaluate whether the stress of the job, or the hereditary makeup of the person, was responsible for premature heart attacks. These countries have twin registries. Thus it was possible to find sets of twins, only one of whom had had a heart attack. In both studies the twin with the attack had worked far more than the standard number of working hours, had assumed a greater responsibility on his job, seldom took more than a half hour for lunch, and occasionally worked on weekends and throughout his vacations. In all cases, the twin with the coronary artery disease had experienced harder mental and physical work. In women with heart disease, the heavier workload was a discriminating factor. All such women held several jobs and had considerably heavier work pressure than their non-affected twin.

Some people think that physical activity protects us from developing coronary artery disease. Dr. Theorell in Sweden attempted to address this question by following over 5000 construction workers for a period of several years. Fifty-one developed a heart attack. The victims had a preponderance of unfavorable work conditions and overwork, suggesting that strenuous physical activity is not completely protective.

Another popular myth links coronary artery disease more with executives than blue collar or clerical workers. Apparently this is not true either. The Framingham Heart Study in Massachusetts followed several hundred women for eight years. Coronary heart disease rates were almost twice as great among women holding clerical jobs compared to housewives (10.6% vs. 5.4%). The most significant predictors of coronary heart disease among clerical women were suppressed hostility, a non-supportive boss, and decreased job mobility. Among working women, clerical workers who had children and were married to blue collar workers were at highest risk of developing coronary heart disease (21%). Apparently, having to hold a job while raising a family in a low income household is extremely stressful.

Other studies also have found a higher frequency of heart attacks in factory workers than in executives. It appears that workers with limited job mobility, and no latitude in decision making, are subject to far more stress than the executive, who is able to delegate some of his responsibilities. It is stressful to work at the same task all day long, particularly when that task is a monotonous one, and the worker has little to say in the work that has to be done.

TYPE A PERSONALITY

A great deal has been written about so-called Type A people being at higher risk for coronary heart disease than Type B people. Type As supposedly have a style of behavior characterized by intense striving for achievement, competitiveness, easily provoked impatience, time urgency, abruptness of gesture or speech, over-commitment to vocation or profession, and excesses of drive and hostility. There is considerable controversy as to whether such behavior exists as an inherent characteristic, or whether it is simply acquired as a result of job related stress. Thus, it may not be the personality that produces the coronary prone behavior, but the stress of the job that creates the personality, and then leads to a heart attack. Because Type A people can be retrained and Type B people may become Type As, these arbitrary characterizations are probably no more than reactions to environmental stress.

Occupational stress has been implicated in almost every important study looking at stress as a major factor in the premature development of heart disease. Unfortunately, most of this information has appeared in medical journals not usually read by heart specialists. As a result, the relationship between emotional stress and heart disease has remained comparatively unknown, and doctors usually don't look at stress when treating patients with known or potential disease.

Indeed, much of the information I have discussed in this chapter is not known to most doctors who see patients with heart problems. One of the purposes of this book is to educate patients so that they are at least as well informed, or even more informed, than their physicians.

HOW TO AVOID DEVELOPING
HEART DISEASE FROM STRESS

Had George Thompson's doctor known of the relationship between emotional stress, high blood pressure, and heart disease, there is no doubt the outcome of his illness would have been different. His blood pressure should have been treated with blood pressure medication and not tranquilizers. The stress at work should have been severely curtailed, and he should have received the beta blocker drug Inderal for both stress and high blood pressure. In fact, his resting blood pressure of 150/90 should not have been accepted by his doctor as his true pressure. It did not reflect what the value would have been at work on a normally stressful day. If George's doctor had treated him better, the heart attack would not have taken place and George would still be president of the company.

How can you, the reader, prevent stress from damaging your heart? Before you attempt to deal with stress, it would be best to determine if you are exhibiting any of its manifestations. Mental signs of stress include a constant sense of urgency, or hurry, never having enough time, nervousness, irritability, short temper, anger, impatience, difficulty concentrating, insomnia, depression, chronic fatigue, weight gain or loss, and unhappiness. Physical manifestations include headaches of both the tension and migraine types, stomach or duodenal ulcers, intermittent diarrhea, an elevated blood pressure, irregular beating of the heart, muscle and joint pains, bouts of asthma, skin rashes, and an increasing dependency upon alcohol. If you have several of these symptoms or physical problems, consider the possibility that you may be under stress.

Stress can be dealt with in several ways. These include avoiding the situations that generate it, using different techniques to reduce the reaction to stress, and using certain drugs to block the effects of stress on the body, particularly, the cardiovascular system.

Avoidance of the effects of stress primarily depends upon identifying the cause. Are you overworked at your job? Reducing your workload, if possible, may help. A daily "to-do" list is often useful. Do you flounder or work inefficiently because you either do not set goals for yourself, or you set unreachable ones? Perhaps you drink eight to ten cups of coffee per day. This would make many people nervous. Unfortunately, it is not always possible to avoid the tension of your job or living situation. Consequently, only a minority of people can deal with their problems this way.

A variety of stress management programs exist. Some consist of taped lectures or seminars, and some can be obtained through individuals such as behavioral psychologists who specialize in this area. These programs emphasize approaches such as specific relaxation techniques, daily exercise, meditation, time management methods, assertiveness techniques and biofeedback. In addition, books have been written about dealing with stress. The breadth of the subject is such that a complete discussion is beyond the scope of this book. Indeed, purchasing one or more books on stress reduction would not be a bad way to start.

By far the most effective drugs for dealing with stress are the beta blockers. The various kinds and how they work will be discussed in later chapters. Students often take beta blockers to neutralize the stress associated with examinations. Speakers who tend to have stage fright have found that Inderal abolishes their fear. These, however, are acute situations. Chronic stress is another matter. As yet, there are no human studies in which the prophylactic administration of a beta blocker has been shown to prevent the development of cardiovascular disease. This is largely because it is not possible to predict who is going to develop high blood pressure or heart disease with complete certainty. Yet, we know that an individual with a strong family history of high blood pressure has a very strong probability of developing hypertension when subjected to chronic stress. Unfortunately, most doctors will not administer a beta blocker to prevent the onset of hypertension, but will give medication once it develops. By then, however, complications may have already developed such as an enlarged heart, or thickening of the muscular walls of blood vessels throughout the body. What, then, should you do? Psychiatrists might prescribe appropriate medication since this problem is partly in their field. Some internists and cardiologists are knowledgeable enough about behavioral medicine to recognize that prevention is more effective than treating a disease after it develops. Finding such a physician may be difficult and require numerous phone calls to physicians' offices or the local medical society to determine who specializes in this area. But you can make changes in your life that will significantly lower your chances of developing heart disease. All it takes is a determination to start; that is always the first step.

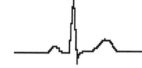

4.

DISCOUNT MEDICINE

How to gamble with your life
and the lives of your family

IN THE PAST FEW YEARS a variety of health care delivery systems have emerged whose purpose is to provide medical care at a lower cost. They go by various names but the most familiar are health maintenance organizations (HMOs), managed health care plans, and preferred provider organizations (PPOs). Actually, HMOs as typified by Kaiser, have existed for over 40 years and only recently have other forms of managed care plans come on to the scene.

Individual plans differ in how they go about controlling the costs of medical care. These differences are becoming increasingly blurred as hybrids evolve. It is far more important for you to understand that the plan you are dealing with, whatever its form, has the goal of controlling the costs of medical care by restricting the benefits. In non-emergency situations, cost control takes precedence over the quality of care offered. It is helpful to understand the basic differences between traditional HMOs and the newer managed health care plans because these differences may influence how you are treated should you become ill.

HMOS

An HMO is one form of a managed health care plan. It differs from the usual managed plan in that the HMO employs its own doctors and they are only allowed to see patients who are members of the HMO. These doctors must obey the rules of the HMO including the number of patients they see each day, how much time can be spent with each one, what diagnostic tests can be ordered, what drugs can be prescribed, and how often the patient may be seen. If referral to a specialist is necessary, it must be to one employed by the HMO. Because as many patients as possible must be seen each day, rarely is there time to perform anything more than a superficial examination. The HMO doctor usually doesn't have the time to answer questions or adequately explain a medical condition to a patient.

In a HMO an individual, or a whole family, will sign up for all medical care in exchange for a flat monthly fee. If the patient is on Medicare, then Medicare pays the fee directly to the HMO and there are usually no additional fees to the patient. In such instances, however, the patient is not covered if he elects to see a physician outside the HMO. When the entire family is covered by the HMO, every member of the family may see a physician without additional charges. Since a variety of specialists, as well as family doctors, are employed by the HMO, the patient does not have to pay for out-of-pocket expenses when referral is necessary. Nor does the patient have to pay for laboratory work. If hospitalization is required, those costs are covered too.

An HMO patient cannot see a specialist without seeing a family practitioner first, and then only if the latter feels it is necessary. Indeed, he may not be allowed to visit a physician at all but may have to see a nurse, nurse-practitioner, physician's assistant or technician for non-life-threatening illness. As a rule he is not able to get an immediate appointment for a non-emergency illness but may have to wait a week or more to see a family doctor, and months to see a specialist. In essence, HMOs ration health care. It a patient is a victim of medical malpractice, he is not allowed to sue but has to agree to binding arbitration by a board that limits the malpractice award.

MANAGED HEALTH CARE PLANS

In contrast, managed health care plans administer health care delivery by fee for service doctors who contract to provide care at greatly discounted rates, often as much as 50% below their regular fees. The patient, or his employer, will contract with the plan and pay it a fixed rate for whatever care the doctor *and the plan* deems necessary. The plan, in turn, reimburses the doctor for those services. In many cases the patient must pay a small but additional co-payment. The doctor is not allowed to bill the patient for the difference between his usual fee and the discounted fee. Although this arrangement may work when both doctor and plan agree on what services should be provided, major problems arise when there is disagreement.

Physicians who contract with a managed care organization are free to see their own private patients, or even to contract with several different plans. Although not employed by the health care plan, they are responsible for all the health care needs of the patients in the plan, even if it fails financially. In certain kinds of managed care plans known as preferred provider organizations (PPOs), no such liability exists on the part of the doctor.

Managed care plans also contract with various hospitals for a discounted fee. The hospital, in turn, will provide bare bones service, that is, whatever is essential, but not one bit more. If a patient is admitted to a hospital that does not have a contract with the plan, the patient's hospitalization will not be covered unless it is a true emergency.

In some managed care plans, the patients and doctors theoretically have more freedom. Patients can select the specialist of their choice and doctors can refer patients to a specialist, provided the doctor is a member of the managed care plan. As a rule, the number of such available specialists is extremely limited.

Unlike an HMO physician who is required to see a certain number of patients a day, a doctor with a contract with a managed care plan can spend as much time as he wishes with a patient.

The problem is that he will not be reimbursed for all that time. Indeed, the fee he receives for a plan patient is so low that in order to make any money he must see as many patients as he can in as short a time as possible. Thus the result is the same—the patient is denied a proper examination.

If extraordinary care, tests or consultations are needed, or if hospitalization or surgery is required, the doctor must first obtain permission from the plan. This could mean a delay of days or weeks, and literally hours of hassle by the physician's staff to get approval. If the doctor does not receive the authorization, the plan will not pay. Managed care plans are notorious for regularly denying such additional services. As a result, many physicians become so frustrated trying to obtain additional medical care for their patients that they give up, or alternatively, never even try. In either case, the result is the same—the managed care plan saves money.

Under the guise of cost control, managed care plans strongly influence how doctors practice medicine, even though the doctor is not an employee. A substantial portion of the physician's practice may be members of a given health plan. In this case, unless the physician cooperates and provides low cost care, he will be dropped as a provider. Since the patients belong to the plan, the doctor will no longer be allowed to see these patients.

WHY DISCOUNT MEDICINE HAS NOT GROWN UNTIL RECENTLY

Prior to the nineties, HMOs were the main type of managed health care plans offering discount medicine. In theory, an HMO sounds like a very attractive idea. Since their inception, this kind of health care delivery has always been able to attract not only individuals, but large groups such as employees from an entire company, unions and other types of organizations.

HMOs have been attractive to doctors as well, particularly new ones. Each doctor is paid a large initial salary, regardless of the number of patients seen, and has liberal vacation benefits, paid time-off for educational meetings, retirement benefits and other perks. He does not have to pay for any professional expenses such as office rent, malpractice insurance and professional fees, all of which can be substantial. In addition, at the end of the year, if there are funds left over, the doctor will receive a bonus.

In spite of what seems to be an attractive system of medical care to patients, and one that is supposedly less costly, discount health care in the form of HMOs was unable to capture more than 10% to 15% of the patient population until just the past few years. With the recent introduction of other forms of discount care, and their emphasis as a cornerstone of health care reform by the Clinton administration, as many as 50% of the population now has some kind of managed care. Yet this increase does not represent an improvement in health care delivery by the discount plans, but is a reflection of the enormous increase in the cost of conventional medical care coupled with the effects of a sagging economy. Companies and individuals have been forced to accept the cheapest form of care available. Nor does the willingness of doctors to engage in discount care mean this is a desirable form of health care delivery. In the past few years we have seen an oversupply of physicians in a poor economy; accordingly many doctors are willing to reduce their fees merely to hold on to their patients.

Prior to the nineties, why didn't HMOs prosper on their own? Why have only a minority of people enrolled as members for so many decades? The primary reason had to do with the restrictions placed upon both doctors and patients. Until recently, HMOs had trouble hiring and keeping doctors. Often a new doctor would become an HMO physician for a short time, and then leave as soon as he found an opportunity in private practice. Few would remain an HMO physician. In addition, HMO doctors were looked down upon by their private practice counterparts, mainly because many private physicians had started their careers working for HMOs and knew first-hand how the system forced doctors to practice poor medicine.

I am convinced HMOs never really took off before the recession because patients were dissatisfied with the quality of care and with the restrictions imposed on them. Groups of patients obtained through industry contracts were constantly getting annoyed with the HMO and leaving. At the same time, new groups would be attracted by the low prices and would join up. Therefore, enrollments stayed at a fairly constant level, but with different patient groups revolving through. The following case history illustrates just a few of the more common problems that are being seen with discount medical care.

A TYPICAL DISCOUNT MEDICAL CARE SCENARIO

Fred Barry was a 45-year old high school English teacher with a wife, two teenage sons and a four-year old daughter. The last addition hadn't been planned but was welcomed and loved by all members of the family. His hospital insurance was coming up for renewal and he had been thinking of trying a different form of insurance. The family had suffered a number of minor illnesses during the past few years and his wife had required an operation. Although everyone had recovered with no complications, his insurance had not covered all the expenses. The insurance carrier was always returning their forms claiming the test or procedure was not covered by their policy. As a result, the Barry family had to pay several hundred dollars each year in doctor expenses. Last year when both he and his wife had been ill, it had cost nearly $1,500.

Fred was thinking about joining an HMO in his area. As a teacher, he had the option of buying private insurance or belonging to an HMO. According to the HMO brochures, a fixed amount each month would cover the entire family for both doctor's visits and hospitalization. They would have no worries about the insurance company refusing coverage and, therefore, they wouldn't have any additional out-of-pocket expenses. Additionally, he and his wife would be eligible for annual physical examinations at no extra cost. The brochure also claimed that the emergency room of the HMO hospital was staffed twenty-four-hours a day; if any member of the family became ill after hours, they would be seen as promptly as possible by medical personnel.

Fred decided to talk to some of his friends who used the HMO to learn how they liked it. A fellow teacher reported using it once when his child broke his arm. Aside from the fact that they had to go back the next day to have the fracture set, after having waited in the emergency room for four hours, he was satisfied—and it hadn't cost him anything.

This should have been a red flag to Fred. The child could have had serious complications if the jagged edge of the bone had cut an artery or injured a nerve; permanent damage might have resulted. It was cheaper to call in the orthopedic consultant during regular office hours rather than in the middle of the night, so the HMO gambled nothing would go wrong.

Another friend said his wife had used the HMO during her last pregnancy. She was not allowed to see her assigned obstetrician until three periods were missed. After that, she was checked by the nurse. He then went on to add that when labor started, his wife was sent home from the hospital twice by the nurse-practitioner because she was not "ready," and during the delivery the doctor had to use forceps. "The baby is O.K. now," he said, "but last month she developed a temperature of 107 degrees and they had to see her in the emergency room. They gave her a shot, and told us how to bring her temperature down at home. Neither the delivery nor the emergency room visit cost me a penny," he added. "And the nurse sees her every three months in the well baby clinic."

This should have been another red flag. During the first two to three months of pregnancy, the fetus is the most vulnerable to developmental defects from accidental exposure to a variety of drugs and environmental toxins. It is wise to counsel any prospective mother as early as possible so she knows what to avoid. Having seen the obstetrician, she did not see him again until she was in the delivery room. Had some complication developed, it would not have been detected until it was too late. For example, there was a very good possibility this mother had some problem that delayed delivery of the child. During the times she was sent home, the baby may well have developed fetal distress resulting in brain damage or even death. That the baby was ultimately delivered by forceps suggests that the mother should have had a Cesarean section. Again, the HMO gambled.

The same baby, when nearly two, developed a high temperature but was sent home with instructions to the parents on how to bring the temperature down. The child not only should have been hospitalized, but probably admitted to the intensive care unit. Had convulsions occurred, she could have died or sustained brain damage. Again the HMO played the odds that her temperature would go down. The parents may not recognize for many years that the high temperature caused brain damage and they have a developmentally slow child.

Fred, unaware the examples cited by his friends were poor medical care, discussed the matter with his wife. They were both swayed by the low monthly cost and the absence of additional costs. Accordingly, they decided to change over to the HMO.

Both Fred and his wife took their annual "physical exams." They filled out questionnaires, had their blood pressures taken, had an electrocardiogram, blood tests, and a urinalysis performed, and Fred's wife had a Pap smear by the nurse. When Fred asked if they would see a doctor, they were told it was not really necessary for routine examinations.

These were not true physical examinations but merely the measurement of some basics. The nurses were efficient, yet it was possible the Barrys might have an abnormality that only a doctor would have detected. However, one of the factors that had encouraged Fred to join the HMO was the promise of an annual physical examination. Was this not a form of fraudulent misrepresentation?

A few months later Fred began having pain while urinating. He called the HMO to request an appointment with a urologist, but was directed to the family clinic instead. He was disappointed the earliest appointment he could get was in one week. Since the pain was not severe at the time, he agreed to wait. At the end of a week, however, he was having considerable discomfort. On the day of his appointment, he sat in the waiting room with twenty other patients for two hours, was finally seen by a nurse, and sent to the laboratory for a urinalysis. There he waited his turn for another hour. When finally seen—briefly, by a general practitioner—he was given a prescription and told to come back if his symptoms failed to disappear. He asked again about seeing a urologist, but was told there was a three month waiting period. Within a week his symptoms went away and he soon forgot the incident.

As time went on, Fred noticed some new symptoms—he was thirsty all the time and was urinating more, although he had no pain. Also, he was eating more but wasn't gaining any weight. He remembered his father had diabetes and had shown similar symptoms. This time Fred tried to get an appointment with an internist at the HMO. Again he was told he would have to be seen first in the family practice clinic, and the next appointment was in three weeks. When finally examined by the family practice doctor, blood tests were obtained and the diagnosis of diabetes was confirmed. Once more he asked about seeing an internist but was told, "It isn't necessary."

Fred was advised to make an appointment with the diabetic clinic where he was taught by a nurse about insulin injections, diet, and how to check his urine. Over the next several months his insulin dosages were adjusted by the diabetic nurse, his symptoms disappeared and he felt fine—and he was pleased that it wasn't costing any extra money.

Two years later, at the time of his so-called annual examination, the nurse mentioned his blood pressure was slightly elevated but not to a level that would require medication. He was teaching another class at school and lately had been under more tension. Fred assumed, therefore, his blood pressure was elevated because of the stress.

One evening, a few months later, while grading some papers, Fred noted some chest pain. Gradually it became worse and simply would not go away. When he called the HMO emergency room, the receptionist said they were very busy and could not see him right away. If he would drive over they would see him when they could. His teenage sons were not home, and his wife was visiting her mother with the youngest child. There was no one to drive him, and he was in too much pain to drive himself. He decided to wait until his wife returned.

When his wife arrived home, one look at her husband convinced her she should send for an ambulance. She called the HMO but was told all their vehicles were out on calls. They would send one as soon as they could. The ambulance didn't arrive for nearly twenty minutes and Fred's pain was getting worse. When Fred arrived at the emergency room, he was brought directly inside by the ambulance attendants and seen about fifteen minutes later by the doctor who ordered an injection for pain. Next, an electrocardiogram, x-ray and blood tests were taken and oxygen started. He was maintained on a monitor and checked at intervals by one of the nurses. Soon his pain began to subside and he felt much better.

One hour later the pain was completely gone; the doctor checked his heart again and informed him that, so far, all the tests were negative. Nevertheless, the doctor wanted the staff cardiologist see him. When the cardiologist arrived he seemed rather arrogant and indifferent. He listened only briefly with a stethoscope, glanced quickly at the electrocardiogram, and stated there didn't seem to be anything wrong with his heart. Fred was to make an appointment with the family practice clinic in about a week.

Fred returned home, but in the following week continued to have occasional episodes of chest pain; however, none was as severe as the original. When seen in the family practice clinic, an electrocardiogram was again taken, and it was still normal. He was told the pains would eventually go away; if the pain persisted he should take aspirin. This information was greeted with relief, for the whole family was to go on vacation the following week to Canada.

Fred never got to Canada. In Seattle his chest pain returned more severe than ever. Fortunately, a large hospital was close to the motel and he went directly to the emergency room. He was seen immediately by the emergency room doctor and within twenty minutes was examined by a cardiologist. This time Fred was hospitalized. Not only did he have a massive heart attack but heart failure as well. Additionally, his blood pressure was found to be very high—over 200, and he had evidence of a chronic kidney infection. He remained in the hospital for two weeks and spent the next three to four months recuperating.

Fred Barry eventually returned to work, but for the rest of his life he will be severely limited because of a damaged heart and kidney. If another heart attack occurs, his chance for survival will be poor. Furthermore, he will remain on medication for both his heart and blood pressure for the rest of his life. His chronic kidney infection will flair up from time to time and require antibiotics. Ultimately, Fred may die many years prematurely from combined kidney and heart disease. Yes, he did save money while he belonged to the HMO, but it cost him his health, and it may cost him his life. At the very least, his medicines over the next several years will cost him many times the amount of money he "saved" by joining the HMO. Furthermore, if he attempts to return to private insurance coverage, his kidney and heart disease, high blood pressure and diabetes all will be excluded as pre-existing conditions!

WHAT WENT WRONG?

What went wrong and how could it have been avoided? To begin with, Fred, although intelligent and a good teacher, was not too knowledgeable about the field of medicine. Like most people, he was unable to distinguish between good and bad medicine. Had he been able to make this distinction, he would have recognized the poor care his friends received at the time of his initial inquiries.

Fred's plight could almost entirely be blamed on the poor care he received over the years at his HMO. Remember the urine infection? He should have seen a urologist then. With proper care and follow up, the doctor could have made sure Fred's infection was completely cured. Because there were no symptoms, it smoldered in his kidneys for years. When Fred was denied permission to see a urologist he lost his freedom of choice. Had his private insurance still been in effect, he could have obtained an appointment with any number of urologists within twenty-four hours. Special tests would have been done to determine the source of his infection, and why it had occurred. His diabetes, which predisposes victims to kidney infections, would have been discovered and treated early instead of late. Yes, such tests are more expensive, and may not be covered by the insurance company. But they are cheaper than the alternative.

The lingering infection damaged Fred's kidneys. This in turn was sufficient to raise his blood pressure above normal. However, the HMO failed to detect this because they didn't take enough readings. If they had diagnosed the elevation in pressure, Fred could have taken drugs to lower it and thereby spared his heart the added strain—the strain that lead directly to his heart attack. He was lucky with the first chest pains, he should have been hospitalized immediately and watched carefully by a cardiologist. Had this been done, in all probability his heart attack could have been avoided.

Why wasn't Fred hospitalized? Did the cardiologist simply make a mistake, or was he guilty of poor judgment? We'll probably never know, but several things could have influenced his judgment. One could have been a lack of hospital beds, which would have meant placing Fred in another hospital at considerable cost to the HMO. Another reason might be the extra work involved in admitting a new patient to the hospital. After all, the HMO-employed cardiologist does not make any more money by putting another patient in the hospital. In fact, he loses money for every patient admitted because it reduces the HMO profits. Finally, the cardiologist simply may have been over-worked with an office full of patients because the HMO saves money by hiring fewer doctors. When Fred's pain disappeared, the cardiologist felt he could avoid hospitalization.

If a patient had an unquestionable heart attack in the situation described, the HMO doctor would have admitted him, and he would have received good care. But in cases in which the diagnosis is in doubt, decisions are often made on the basis of what is best for the HMO rather than what is good for the patient. The

HMO gambles. If the patient recovers, as they often do, then they have saved a considerable amount of money. If they lose the gamble, the HMO loses very little, but the patient may lose his health or his life.

Fred's case brings up a host of other questions too. Why couldn't he see an internist for his diabetes? Why was this condition only treated by a nurse? Why did he have to wait to see the family practice doctor? Why did he never see a doctor regarding his blood pressure? Why wasn't an ambulance sent immediately when he had chest pains?

The answer to all these questions is financial. It costs more to pay a specialist than a diabetic nurse. It costs more to hospitalize a patient than to treat that person at home. It costs more for a doctor to do annual examinations than nurses. It costs more to hire several urologists rather than one. It also costs more to hire extra family practitioners so the patients do not have to wait as long to be seen. When the overall cost of medical care is reduced, then cheaper "health care" can be offered to the public who receive the "benefits."

When cheaper health care is offered, larger numbers of patients and employee groups will join the HMO. Typically, additional doctors are not hired—the available doctors simply have to see extra patients. All this means greater profits for the HMO. Since the doctors share in those profits, it follows that the less that can be done for every patient, the more profit the doctor makes. As a consequence, he is not rewarded for practicing good medicine, he is rewarded for practicing poor medicine!

HOW DISCOUNT MEDICAL CARE PLANS ATTRACT PATIENTS

Discount medical care plans attract new members by making claims that they can offer the same quality of medical care as doctors in private practice but at a much lower cost. The quality of care is good, they state, because they hire only the best doctors. This is a subtle form of deceptive advertising because it is misleading. Yes, they may hire good doctors, and those doctors are capable of practicing good medicine—but most of the time they are limited because of the restrictions imposed by the system. With few exceptions, these doctors are overworked because of the large numbers of patients they must see each day. The situation is not unlike teaching a class of children. With only 10 or 12 children in each class, the teacher is able to give each one the individual attention needed. Increase the number in the class to 35 or 40, and the learning falls off dramatically. If a physician can only spend a few minutes with each patient, he can't possibly do as good a job as he would normally. In many instances it may not matter, because the patient is doing well, and really doesn't need to be seen. But most of the time, particularly with heart patients, their disease progresses silently. The patient will exhibit few clues and they are not easy to detect. In other words, it will take time for the doctor to find them. But time is the one thing these physicians don't have. The clue will be missed, the patient's disease will progress, a complication will occur, damage will befall his heart, and his life will be shortened. If the patient dies, his death will be attributed to heart disease rather than the negligence of the plan. One can die very cheaply this way.

Discount groups advertise that their rate of hospitalization is much lower than doctors in private practice. This claim is true. What they do not tell you is that this neat trick is accomplished by denying admission to many patients that really should be in a hospital. Not hospitalizing the patient costs them less money and they can offer cheaper medical care. In addition, it is well known that discount plans tend to "skim" patients. In other words, they tend to take only younger and healthier patients who are less likely to become ill and need hospitalization.

LOW COST HEALTH CARE MAY BE THE MOST EXPENSIVE

It should be evident that discount medicine, regardless of the form it takes, penalizes both the patient and the doctor. It penalizes the patient by reducing the quality of medical care offered, and takes away his freedom in selecting the doctor or specialist of his choice. At the same time the patient is mislead into believing high quality medical care is being offered at a lower price.

That is deception. When the consumer is forced to accept a lower quality product because the cost is less, he loses his freedom.

Discount medicine also penalizes patients in a less obvious way. When hospitals offer their services to discount medical groups at steep discounts, their losses have to be made up in other ways. Typically they practice cost shifting. If, for example, the cost of using an operating room for bypass surgery is $2,000 and they have contracted to charge a managed health plan only $1,000, they recoup that loss by increasing the cost to the regular patient with standard insurance to $3,000. This of course, drives up the cost of hospitalization insurance. Discount medicine doesn't really save money, it merely passes the costs on to someone else.

The physician is the second innocent victim of discount medicine. Not only has the patient lost his freedom of choice as to whom he sees, but the physician has also. He has little control over the number of patients he must see each day, or to whom he can refer a patient for consultation. He must use another discount group physician whether he thinks him capable or not. Good doctors are concerned not only about the quality of medical care they themselves render to their patients, but also about the quality of care given by other doctors who see their patient.

If both doctors and patients are dissatisfied with HMOs and other forms of discount medicine, how can they possibly flourish? One reason is simply that many people cannot afford any other medical care. To the poor person who is barefooted, a cheap pair of shoes is better than nothing at all. Also, many people are covered as a condition of their employment. The employer, or his chief financial officer, is not concerned with the quality of care, only its cost. Since discount plans offer less expensive care than private insurance plans, it is the plan that the employer picks. The employer doesn't recognize that in the long run, the poor quality care will result in more time lost from the job and poorer performance as a result of his employees' ill health.

These kinds of plans will continue to thrive until the public becomes informed, and learns to recognize the dangers of cut-rate medical care. By and large, we get what we pay for, whether it is a car or a doctor. To be sure, the current system of the private practice of medicine has many faults including a very high cost; and clearly there are too many tests and too many surgeries done today. Like a democracy, it is a poor system; but is there anything better around? I believe that the various forms of discount medicine are no better. Instead they are a constant source of danger to the unsuspecting, sick, vulnerable and captive patient. Above all, they are not cheaper! They cost the public more by failing to deliver quality care and by forcing hospitals and doctors to shift part of the burden on to private and insured patients. The public must learn that in the long run the most costly medical care is actually the so-called cheapest medical care. Private medicine may be guilty of too much, too soon, but the public should know that discount medicine will mean too little, too late.

WHAT YOU CAN DO TO PREVENT
DENIAL OF HEALTH CARE SERVICES

Despite my concerns about the quality of medical care you may receive in a managed care plan, I realize that millions of people are enrolled in such services. And, if you receive this care through your employer, there is probably little you can do about changing it once enrolled. This section will help you negotiate your way through your plan and encourage you to take action to force it to work for your own advantage.

Rarely is a patient knowledgeable enough about his own disease to know what tests should be ordered, or what treatment should be rendered. Some patients have acquired such information painfully through long experience with their conditions. Obviously you do not want to wait until you have had multiple attacks of the same disease to learn about it—by then it may be too late. The best way to obtain the information you need is through reading about your condition.

Go to the library or your neighborhood bookstore. Find out as much as you can about your medical condition, whether it is a heart problem or some other disease. There are enough reference books and textbooks available to provide you with at least the basic knowledge. Nobody should do this for you; you must take the responsibility yourself, unless your illness prevents it. When you find out about your disease, what its causes are, what other medical conditions aggravate it, how it is diagnosed, what tests are used, and how it should be treated, then you will have the ammunition to deal with the doctors at your health care plan. In addition, you will know enough to talk with the paramedical people who try to limit your access to the doctor, and to the administrators who run your health plan, and who have the final decision on what the doctor is allowed to do. If you cannot obtain the information through the library or bookstore, call the medical society in the city you live. It may already have information pamphlets on the very condition you have. If it is a heart problem, call your local heart association and ask for information brochures. If written material is unavailable, obtain the name of a good specialist from a friend or the medical society. Set up an appointment for a consultation. Let the doctor's receptionist know that you do not wish to undergo any tests or treatment, but that you would like his advice on whether the health plan you belong to has diagnosed and treated your condition properly. In other words, are they denying you necessary health care services? You will have to pay for such a consultation yourself; however, since you are not asking the doctor to do any tests or treat you, the cost should be reasonable. And, it may be the best money you ever spend.

If you determine that your medical problem has not been handled in an appropriate way, request to see your treating doctor. Politely tell him that you are aware that he has failed to diagnose and/or treat you in the usual and customary manner, that you do not feel you have received proper medical attention, and you are requesting that he correct the problem. If he can do it himself, this may be perfectly adequate. However, if you feel it is essential for you to be referred to a specialist, then insist upon it. You are a consumer, and you have certain rights. Make it clear to the doctor that you have joined his managed health care plan under the assumption that the quality of medical care was equal to that provided by doctors in private practice. If you feel that the

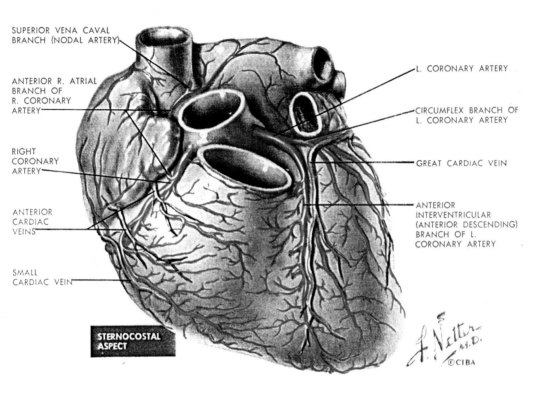

SUPERIOR VENA CAVAL
BRANCH (NODAL ARTERY)

ANTERIOR R. ATRIAL
BRANCH OF
R. CORONARY
ARTERY

RIGHT
CORONARY
ARTERY

ANTERIOR
CARDIAC
VEINS

SMALL
CARDIAC VEIN

L. CORONARY ARTERY

CIRCUMFLEX BRANCH OF
L. CORONARY ARTERY

GREAT CARDIAC VEIN

ANTERIOR
INTERVENTRICULAR
(ANTERIOR DESCENDING)
BRANCH OF L.
CORONARY ARTERY

STERNOCOSTAL
ASPECT

©CIBA

FIGURE 1. The coronary arteries on the surface of the heart as they are usually depicted. This is the image the cardiologist visualizes when he thinks of the coronary circulation. Note how the arteries branch like a tree, and that there appears to be no connections between the right and left coronary systems. Only a limited number of such branches can be followed because the artery enters the heart muscle and disappears from view. (Abbreviations: R:right; L:left.) *(Reprinted with the permission of the Ciba-Geigy Pharmaceutical Company from the Ciba Collections of Medical Illustrations by Netter, F.H., Summit, N.J. 1969.)*

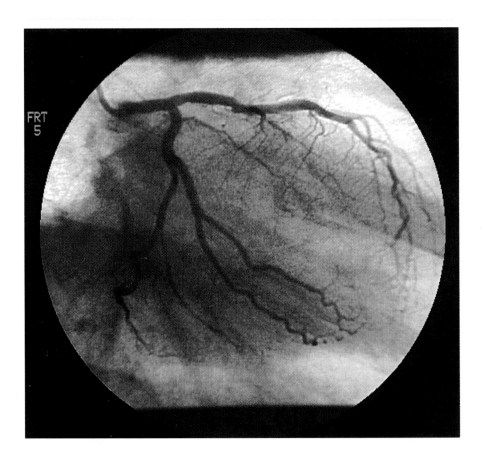

FIGURE 2. The angiogram. By injecting dye that is opaque to x-rays into a coronary artery at its origin, and taking pictures with a high speed camera, the inside or lumen of the artery becomes visible. Even though the lumen of the artery may be seen through the heart muscle, note there are relatively few branches. This is because the resolution of the angiographic technique is such that vessels smaller than 0.5 millimeter cannot be seen. As noted in Figure 1, there appears to be no connecting vessels between the major branches. Compare with Fig. 3.

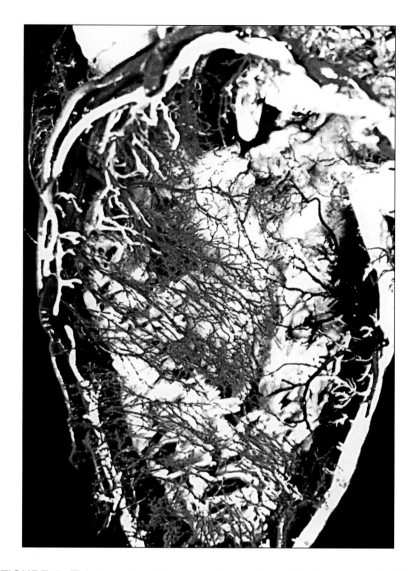

FIGURE 3. This is a heart from a 17-year-old male. It was created by injecting red-colored vinylite into the left coronary system, blue vinylite into lthe right coronary system, and white vinylite into the coronary venous system. The heart muscle was then dissected away. Observe the extensive network of small vessels not depicted in Figure 1. Nor are they visualized in Figure 2 because they are too small to be imaged by the angiographic technique. Note there are numerous connecting vessels joining one area of the heart with another. These are called anastomoses, and they, too, are usually invisible on an angiogram. If an artery becomes narrowed or obstructed, new blood vessels will bud out upstream from the obstruction and will anastomose to a nearby healthy artery. Alternatively, they will reinsert into the mother artery downstream from the obstruction. See text for further details. *(Reprinted with permission of Harper & Row, from James.[2])*

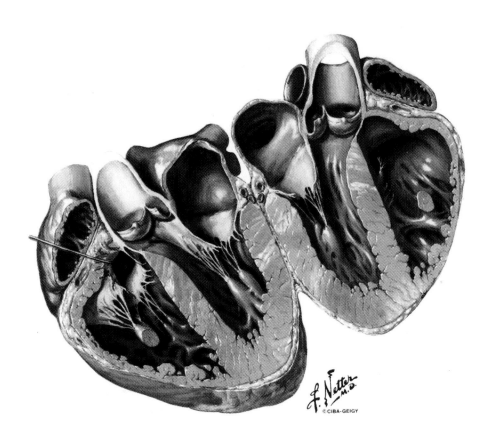

FIGURE 4. A cut section through the heart showing its chambers and its muscular walls. Try to visualize the network of small blood vessels seen in Figure 3 lying within the muscular walls of the heart, and how pressure inside the heart's chambers can be transmitted to within those muscular walls. *(Reprinted with the permission of the Ciba-Geigy Pharmaceutical Company from the Ciba Collections of Medical Illustrations by Netter, F.H., Summit, N.J. 1969)*

care rendered to you was inadequate, say so! Insist, demand that you receive the tests or treatment you feel are necessary. Tell the doctor that if you have a complication of your illness because of inadequate care, he, personally, will be held responsible. If you are forceful enough, and are sure of your information, he will agree to your demands, especially if he knows you are right.

Suppose he refuses, or denies the necessity of your requests. What do you do then? If your health plan is provided by your employer, your most likely chance of success is to go directly to the person in your company who was responsible for setting up the contract with the managed health care plan. He can deal directly with the plan's administrator. When the administrator realizes that he is dealing with the individual who controls whether the company continues to use the plan, you will get cooperation. Count on it. When you push the right button, you will get a response. You, as a lay person, can get more action when there has been wrongful health care services denial than the doctor. The administrator will say "no" to the doctor. He saves money by saying "no." That's his job. Keep in mind that the very definition of a managed health care plan or HMO is one in which emphasis is placed on controlling health care costs. Quality of medical care is a secondary consideration—to them, not to you. On the other hand, if the denial of a test, treatment, or visit to a specialist is going to cost more money in the long run because the plan will lose patients, you are likely to receive cooperation.

Suppose you have joined the managed care plan as an individual, and you have no large company or group to fight for you, what do you do then? Call your local county medical society and talk to their staff. If you have truly been treated improperly, the medical society may be able to intercede for you. They can exert pressure on both the health plan administrator and the doctor.

There is still one other course of action you can take. If the previous recommendations fail, go to a private physician and ask for whatever tests you feel are necessary. If they are negative, you will probably have to pay for the cost yourself, but at least you will know you do not have more serious disease. If the tests are positive, and you do have something wrong that the managed health care plan doctor missed, take the bills to the health plan administrator. Tell them they have to pay the costs or you will send a formal complaint to the insurance commissioner of your state. That should get some action!

Part II:

OVERDIAGNOSIS

and

OVERTREATMENT

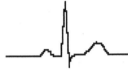

5.

THE CHOLESTEROL DECEPTION

What you've been told about cholesterol
and heart disease may not be true.

IN RECENT YEARS, both the public and physicians alike have been victims of a medical and media blitz about the close relationship between blood cholesterol levels and heart disease. It may come as somewhat of a shock to learn that much, if not most of the information about cholesterol that we have been deluged with, has been distorted to make these conclusions appear true. Scientific data that shows only a weak relationship between cholesterol and heart disease has been deliberately manipulated, and statistical relationships twisted, to make our cholesterol level appear much more important than it really is.

We have been led to believe that an elevated cholesterol level means our coronary arteries will clog with cholesterol plaques, thereby obstructing the flow of blood to the heart muscle, and raising our risk of a heart attack. We are further told that even if we have no evidence of heart disease, we should lower our cholesterol with diet or drug therapy, in order to diminish our likelihood of a heart attack. Finally we have been advised that all of us should live on a low fat, low cholesterol diet, whether we are eight or eighty years old.

Information tending to support the cholesterol theory has been ballyhooed with media hype reminiscent of the opening of a major movie. Any medical article supporting the importance of cholesterol to heart disease is systematically fed to every available lay and medical publication, the wire services, television, and radio for months. In contrast, articles that do not support the cholesterol theory are published once, receive almost no publicity, are ignored and soon forgotten. Never has a medical theory received such vast publicity for so many years, with so little scientific evidence to document it.

WHO BENEFITS FROM THE CHOLESTEROL CAMPAIGN?

Who might benefit the most from the public's fear of elevated cholesterol levels, and how has critical information been distorted to fuel that fear? Because the cholesterol campaign has been so extensive and prolonged, and because an undertaking of such magnitude must require an enormous expenditure of funds, one can deduce there has to be a self-serving reason somewhere. It is safe to assume that reason has to be an economic one.

For starters, a number of pharmaceutical companies manufacture very expensive cholesterol-lowering drugs. In some instances, the cost to the patient can be over $100 per month. Such companies stand to make billions of dollars if both doctors and the public alike can be convinced that it is unhealthy to have a high cholesterol level. In addition, many food companies now market low cholesterol products. Fear of foods containing high amounts of cholesterol will encourage the consumer to purchase the low cholesterol brands. The massive publicity that cholesterol receives makes sense when one realizes that this creates a market for drugs to lower our cholesterol when it's elevated and for foods to keep it from rising.

Evidence to support the cholesterol theory of heart disease is so flimsy that it seems almost incredible so many people (including physicians) have accepted it with conviction. In the fifties, sixties and seventies many studies attempted to prove the relationship between cholesterol and heart disease with little success. These scientific studies had no media hype to support them. Thus, few physicians were swayed by the evidence and the public even less so.

In the eighties, the cholesterol campaign was started in an attempt to convince us through the media what scientific studies could not. To make such a campaign effective, data originating from scientific studies was manipulated to make it appear believable. With modern marketing techniques, adequate funding, and an orchestrated publicity campaign, all but the illiterate were persuaded.

So successful has been the cholesterol campaign that low cholesterol diets are advised for everyone, even though none of the modern studies were done with diet alone, and none involved women or individuals above the age of 60. Surprisingly, even growing children have been advised to reduce their cholesterol intake without regard to potential harmful effects on their special nutritional needs. We don't even have any information supporting the theory that a low cholesterol diet will benefit anyone above the age of 60. In fact, as we shall see, the weak relationship between cholesterol and heart disease hasn't been shown to apply to women of any age.

HOW CHOLESTEROL STUDIES HAVE
BEEN MISREPRESENTED

What is the evidence to support the cholesterol theory, how have studies been misrepresented to make the relationship between cholesterol and heart disease seem more important than it really is, and why was it done? The original evidence became apparent after World War II when a decrease in cardiovascular deaths was noted following wartime food shortages. Subsequently, population studies established that cultures with a low cholesterol intake not only had low blood cholesterol levels, but also a low incidence of heart disease. Since cholesterol was an ingredient of the arteriosclerotic plaques that lined the arterial

walls, eager scientists were only too quick to assume that cholesterol caused heart attacks.

Glossed over was the fact that although differences exist when
one population is compared to another, those differences disappear when people within a population are compared to one another. For example, the Japanese show marked differences in fat
intake, blood cholesterol levels and the incidence of heart disease
when compared to Americans. But when the Japanese are compared to other Japanese, or Americans to Americans, a consistent
relationship cannot be found between dietary intake of fat, cholesterol levels and heart disease. In other words, within a population group, the level of cholesterol has no predictability as to the
likelihood of a heart attack. In fact, far more people with normal
cholesterol levels have heart attacks than those with elevated
cholesterols.[1]

Those convinced that cholesterol kills cite studies showing that
individuals from cultures with a low frequency of heart disease
suffer more heart attacks when they migrate to urban areas and
consume foods high in cholesterol. This assumes that such a move
precipitates changes in diet alone whereas everything changes—
an individual's job, home, level of physical activity, smoking hab-
its, the amount of stress in his life and even his use of leisure
time.

It should not be surprising that the amount of heart disease
found in a population also shows a correlation with sugar and
wine consumption, income level, the number of cigarettes smoked,
the level of stress, the number of television sets in a home, the
number of cars owned, and even the frequency with which silk
stockings are worn.[2] Consequently, a mere association between
cholesterol intake and the frequency of heart disease is insufficient. We need other forms of confirming evidence to be truly
convinced that a causative link exists.

Another little known fact ignored by the cholesterol adherents
is that fat consumption has increased two to four times in countries like Japan, Israel and Switzerland, yet the frequency of heart
disease has dropped markedly in these same countries. Con-

versely, the Chinese eat a low cholesterol diet but suffer a high incidence of coronary artery disease.

One of the most frequent lines of evidence cited by the cholesterol supporters came from animal studies. Certain animals, when fed diets high in cholesterol, develop a form of arteriosclerosis which could be reversed with low cholesterol diets. Claims that such experiments supported the diet-cholesterol theory were riddled with flaws. For example, blood cholesterol levels required to produce arteriosclerosis in rabbits were many times higher than were seen in humans—in some cases as much as twenty times higher. As a result, the development of arteriosclerotic plaques in rabbits was not at all like that seen in humans. In addition, neither the location nor the distribution of such plaques resembled that seen in man. In rabbits, plaques were found in the pulmonary vessels—those vessels going to the lungs. In humans, such a distribution is never found except in rare patients with both congenital heart defects and an elevated pressure in the pulmonary vessels. Also, complications from the presence of arteriosclerosis in rabbits were different from those seen in men.

Experimental arteriosclerosis has been produced with high cholesterol diets in other animals, including primates such as chimpanzees and baboons. Again, as in rabbits, the lesions produced are more similar to a form of fat storage disease rather than human type arteriosclerosis. It is worth mentioning that severe arteriosclerosis has been produced in primates on a cholesterol-free diet merely by subjecting them to environmental stress. On a parallel note, the South American ostrich, the rhea, lives on a cholesterol free, vegetarian diet. Nevertheless, the rhea develops severe arteriosclerosis when forced to live in the stressful confines of a zoo. In short, experimental arteriosclerosis as produced in animals, is simply not the same disease as occurs in man.

THE LIPID RESEARCH CLINIC'S
PRIMARY PREVENTION TRIAL

In 1984 the thrust of the cholesterol campaign changed with the release of a multicenter report from the Lipid Research Clinic's Primary Prevention Trial.[3,4] The study involved 3,606 men for a

mean of 7.4 years. Approximately half were treated with both
diet and a cholesterol-lowering agent known as cholestyramine.
The remainder were treated with a placebo. Statements released
to the press at the time claimed that for the first time it had been
"proven" that lowering cholesterol would reduce the mortality
from heart disease, and lower the risk of having a heart attack. In
a manner reminiscent of a baseball team that had won its first
pennant in 40 years, the cholesterol supporters gloated—or so it
seemed.

Never did a single medical article get so much press for so long.
What made it worse, and even lent it some authenticity, was the
fact that the release of information originated from the National
Heart and Lung Institute, since it was their funds that had supported the study. Little attention was given to the fact that nine
large-scale clinical trials had been conducted previously in Norway, Finland, Australia, England, and the United States with dietary control of cholesterol intake. In these studies over 11,000
patients were studied for periods ranging from 2 to 10 years, and
cholesterol reductions of 7% to 16 % were seen. However, in most
of these studies there was an insignificant decrease in the incidence of coronary artery disease, and no effect on overall mortality of the people studied.[5-8] In other words, lowering cholesterol
levels didn't prevent heart attacks or keep people alive any longer.

The Lipid Research Clinic's Primary Prevention Trial Study
claimed that in the 1,906 men treated with cholestyramine, a significant decrease in cholesterol was attained, along with a 24 %
decrease in mortality from heart disease when compared to the
control group treated with a placebo. If this were true, it indeed
would be important support for the cholesterol theory of heart
disease. It is worth looking at how this study was structured to
understand the actual results.

HOW THE LIPID RESEARCH CLINIC'S PRIMARY
PREVENTION TRIAL WAS DISTORTED

To begin with, the total cost of the Lipid Research Clinic's Primary Prevention Trial Study was approximately $150 million. It
involved a total of 3,806 men. However, the men selected were

not representative of the population at large. They were between the ages of 35 and 59, free of heart disease, and had a high blood cholesterol level that was independent of their diet. There were no women in the study, no patients with heart disease, and no older patients. In order to obtain these subjects, 480,000 individuals had to be screened. Thus, less than one individual out of 126 qualified—hardly a representative sample.

Much of what we hear today about diet and heart disease is based upon this notorious landmark study, therefore it is relevant to review what was said by other medical scientists at that time. Drs. Vitale and Ross,[9] in a critique of this study, stated: "The whole story of the Lipid Research Clinic's Coronary Primary Prevention Trial is an impressive example of misconstrued research results." They suggested that men meeting the screening requirements had a rare form of hypercholesterolemia (high blood cholesterol) and, as such, they represented less than 1% of the general population. Vitale and Ross theorized that this is a unique genetic defect with a clear association between the blood levels of cholesterol and coronary heart disease. Thus, any conclusions drawn from the responses of patients with this rare form of hypercholesterolemia must to be limited to only other patients with the same type of disorder. Any attempt to generalize the findings to the remainder of the population, to women, and especially children was not only unscientific but dishonest.

The Lipid Research Clinic's Primary Prevention Trial Study was not solely a diet study, it was a drug study. The drug used was cholestyramine, a cholesterol-lowering agent, and it was administered to each person in the test group, along with a low cholesterol diet. Because of the design of the study no conclusions can be reached about whether lowering dietary cholesterol would have helped prevent heart disease. If diet alone had been studied, it is extremely unlikely the results would have been any different from all the previous studies which clearly demonstrated that the effect of diet on the incidence of heart attacks was virtually zero.

The real distortion of the results of the study was in the claim of a 24% reduction in the risk of cardiovascular deaths in the test group. Actually, there were 38 deaths from heart disease in the control group and 30 deaths in the cholestyramine treated group during the 7.4 years the patients were studied. Thus, 2.0% of the control group died vs. 1.6% of the cholestyramine treated patients—a net difference of only 0.4 % over a period of more than seven years! This hardly could be considered a significant difference. Furthermore, no actual difference in total overall mortality occurred between the two groups because of an increase in deaths from accidents, violence and cancer in the control group.

To view these results from a slightly different perspective, if 200 people with a high blood cholesterol were to go on a low cholesterol diet for seven years, and take an expensive cholesterol-lowering drug with a high incidence of side effects (68%), less than one out of 200 might benefit at the end of seven years. This benefit, however, would be offset by the increased likelihood of dying from an accident, violence or cancer!

The Lipid Research Clinic's Primary Prevention Trial Study also claimed that the cholestyramine-diet treated patients experienced a 19% reduction in the risk of a nonfatal heart attack. Once again, the actual numbers reveal a statistical distortion. There were 158 nonfatal heart attacks in the placebo treated patients, for a total incidence of 8.3% (1.1% a year). In the cholestyramine treated patients, there were a total of 130 nonfatal heart attacks during the 7.4 years of the study, for a total incidence of 6.8% (0.9% a year). Thus, the total difference in nonfatal heart attacks between those treated, compared to those who were not treated, was only 1.5% over a period of 7.4 years, or only 0.2% per year, and not 19%. In other words, if 100 people took an expensive drug with many side effects for five years, only one might benefit. Clearly, such a difference could occur as a result of chance alone.

In spite of their claims to the contrary, the results of the Lipid Research Clinic's Primary Prevention Trial Study were not significantly different from the nine large-scale clinical trials conducted previously which showed an insignificant decrease in the incidence of coronary artery disease between groups on the basis of cholesterol levels, and no effect on overall mortality.

The investigators in the Lipid Research Clinic's Coronary Primary Prevention Trial made a point of *not* emphasizing that 11 cases of gastrointestinal cancer with 1 death occurred in the placebo group, while the experimental group experienced 21 cases of gastrointestinal cancer and 8 deaths. The total death rate due to cancer in the cholestyramine treated patients was 11/1000. In contrast, the total death rate due to cancer in the United States is only 2/1000—a 5-fold increase. In addition, researchers found a major difference in the incidence of deaths due to accidents, suicides and homicides between the two groups with 11 such deaths in the treated group but only 4 in the placebo group.

It is of interest that the Lipid Research Clinic's investigators left no stone unturned in their manipulation of the data so that insignificant results could be transformed into what appeared to be significant results. Because this was a major government-sponsored study of heroic cost, the design of the study was published in 1979—five years before the results were known.[10] In the beginning they planned to study two primary outcomes: one was to be coronary heart disease related deaths, and the second was to be nonfatal heart attacks. Furthermore, the level at which these events were to be considered significant was what researchers call the 1% level. These separate outcomes are common to all trials because they are easily distinguished—there is nothing questionable about a heart attack or death. Yet, the Lipid Research Clinic's investigators arbitrarily changed the multiple outcomes to a single one of combined coronary heart disease related deaths and nonfatal heart attacks. They also lowered the level of clinical significance to a 5% level. A 5% level of significance is much weaker because it signifies that the results of a study can occur just by chance 5 times out of 100 rather than 1 time out of 100 as with a 1% level of significance. Had the original outcomes and statistical evaluations been used as promised in 1979, I suspect the data could not have been manipulated in any fashion to make the results appear significant.

HOW ARTERIOSCLEROSIS CAN BE
"REVERSED" WITH DRUGS

The second major study the proponents of the cholesterol theory of heart disease use was published just a few years ago. It originated from the University of Southern California in Los Angeles.[11] In this study, 162 men aged 40 to 59 who had previous coronary artery bypass surgery were placed on two cholesterol-lowering drugs, as well as a low cholesterol diet. They received coronary angiograms before the study and again after two years. The claim was made that for the first time regression of arteriosclerosis could be demonstrated. Once again, we began to see large numbers of articles in both the medical and lay press with headlines proclaiming the cholesterol theory of heart disease had now been "proven" with conclusive facts.

In fact, examination of an image of an angiogram from this study which claimed there was less coronary artery narrowing after treatment, showed unequivocal rotation of the position of the patient between the two angiograms taken at two year intervals. Thus the "improvement" may have been nothing more than an illusion created by altering the angle of view in the angiogram. How rotation of the subject's position can influence the appearance of coronary artery narrowing can be demonstrated by squeezing a drinking straw in the middle. If the straw is placed several feet away so that any three dimensional effect is lost, in one view the narrowing will be readily seen. If the straw is now rotated 90 degrees, it will no longer appear narrowed. Similarly, a coronary artery that appears narrowed in one view may appear normal if the patient is turned or rotated so that the x-ray image is viewed from a slightly different angle.

Let's give the authors of this study the benefit of the doubt, and assume their claims were true. Regression was found to occur in only 16.2% of the patients treated, while 2.4% of the untreated patients showed similar improvement. Thus, only 13.8% of the patients in the experimental group achieved any benefit over a two year period. In spite of this so-called benefit, there was no overall difference in cardiovascular events between the two groups. However, a marked difference was seen between the two groups in terms of side effects from medication, with those effects occurring in over 90% of the treated patients.

THE HELSINKI STUDY

Another recent article claiming a beneficial effect from lowering cholesterol was reported in the *New England Journal of Medicine* a few years ago—the so-called Helsinki Study.[12] That work was a five-year trial with 4,081 middle-aged men from 40 to 55-years old, with elevated cholesterol levels and no symptoms. Approximately half received a cholesterol-lowering drug known as gemfibrozil, while the remainder received a placebo. A significant reduction in cholesterol levels and a 34% decrease in mortality among the men taking the gemfibrozil were reported.

Again and again, the data were fed to every medical publication and the lay media. The statistic "34% decrease in mortality" was given banner headlines. Once more, let's look at the actual numbers to see how the 34% was derived.

A total of 11 cardiac deaths occurred in the gemfibrozil patients and 12 in the placebo treated patients at the end of 5 years. A total of 2.7 cardiovascular events (death or non-fatal heart attack) were measured per 100 gemfibrozil treated patients and 4.1 events in the placebo treated patients. Thus, there was only a 1.4% difference between the treated and untreated groups (4.1% vs. 2.7%) over a total period of 5 years. How was the figure 34% arrived at? Simple arithmetic: 1.4% difference between the groups divided by 4.1% events in the placebo group equals 34%! In actuality, this is a percent of a percent and to report it as the major finding is deliberately misleading.

To clarify, a comparison could be made to a rise in the prime lending interest rate from 9% to 10%. When this occurs, one can anticipate headlines that state, "Prime rate goes up 1%." Imagine the confusion that would be generated if the headlines were to state, "Prime rate goes up 11%". Using the Helsinki paper's method of calculation: 1% divided by 9% equals 11%!

WHY CARDIAC SYMPTOMS CAN BE RELIEVED
BY LOW CHOLESTEROL DIETS

Cholesterol evangelists claim that a low fat, low cholesterol diet benefits patients with heart disease and helps relieve their symptoms. The best known of these programs has been the Pritikin diet. When Pritikin was still alive, he claimed that coronary heart disease patients in whom bypass surgery was recommended would improve enough on this diet so they would no longer need surgery. Interestingly enough, what Pritikin claimed was true—patients did have a relief of their symptoms and very definitely could exercise more. Of course the same thing must have been noted during World War II on the grossly deficient diets of that time.

What Pritikin and others overlooked, or ignored, was that such diets are extremely low in calories and anyone adhering to such a program for any length of time, invariably loses a significant amount of weight. Along with the weight loss there is a reduction in fluid intake and frequently in blood pressure. This combination can be successful in achieving a marked decrease in the heart's workload. Reducing the workload is like decreasing one's expenses—one has more money left over. Thus, any reduction in workload on the heart will increase the blood flow to the heart muscle, and have a beneficial influence on the patient's symptoms. Because the public is not knowledgeable about such information, it is easy to see how the claims about the effects of a low cholesterol diet on symptoms of heart disease can be misinterpreted.

It is worth mentioning here that cholesterol is a natural product of the body. Its nucleus is a steroid—the same type of substance that makes up cortisone. Indeed, cholesterol plays a vital role in the formation of cortisone and other hormones. It also plays an important role in digestion. For example, the liver produces approximately 1.5 grams of cholesterol a day while other organs produce about 0.5 gram. This naturally produced cholesterol is several times the amount ingested in the diet. Cholesterol is so necessary to the appropriate function of the body that if the diet is deficient in cholesterol, the liver and other organs will increase their manufacture of the substance to ensure an adequate supply. Apparently this interference with the production of cholesterol by cholesterol-lowering agents is the cause of one of the well known side effects of these drugs, an increase in the formation of gallstones and gall bladder colic. Surgery for gall bladder disease is not without considerable risk and side effects.

HOW FEAR OF HEART DISEASE CAN BE CREATED

The National Cholesterol Education Campaign has arbitrarily declared a cholesterol level above 200 is abnormal. Most industrialized nations use a figure of 250. Countless patients with cholesterol levels between 201 and 250 have been frightened by doctors when told their cholesterol was elevated and that they were thereby at increased risk of a heart attack. Few of these victims are aware that a random cholesterol determination is quite inaccurate and subject to wide variations. For example, emotional stress, age, disease, the seasons and diet can cause extensive fluctuations in normal values. As a result, there is no simply defined normal value. These facts are skillfully ignored by those who are responsible for the cholesterol campaign. By declaring 200 to be the danger threshold rather than 250, they frightened millions more into purchasing cholesterol-lowering drugs and low cholesterol foods.

Not only is the public misled by all this misinformation, but physicians are too. At first glance it may seem that even if a physician recommends a low cholesterol diet, it can't harm the patient. If the patient in question is grossly overweight, this is certainly true. Unfortunately, similar recommendations are often made to elderly patients who are painfully underweight. Such individuals simply do not eat enough food. To advise them to go on a low calorie diet and to simultaneously deprive them of cheap, yet nutritious sources of protein such as eggs, is simply poor judgment.

In many instances I have seen patients with recurring chest pain who have been advised by their doctors to undergo coronary artery bypass surgery. An examination of their medication program usually reveals one, and sometimes two, costly cholesterol-lowering agents that they take daily. Yet, drugs that are effective in eliminating their chest pain have not been prescribed. Clearly, both doctor and patient alike have been duped into believing that lowering cholesterol will lower the likelihood of a heart attack.

Our English speaking cousins and the rest of the world feel differently. Perhaps vested interests overseas have not influenced medical scientists with grant funds and expense-paid trips to lecture at symposia. They have correctly pointed out that if one were to rigidly restrict his dietary intake of fat and cholesterol for his entire life, that person might be able to prolong his life from a few days to a few months.

On October 9-10, 1990, a National Heart, Lung and Blood Institute Conference was held[13] to discuss the relationship between mortality and blood cholesterol levels. Representatives from the United States, Europe, Israel and Japan reviewed studies on 68,406 deaths. They found that people with low cholesterols (below 160 mg, both male and female) had a 20% higher death rate from cancer as well as a 40% higher death rate from non cardiac, non cancer deaths. This latter death rate included a 35% increase in injury deaths, a 15% increase in respiratory deaths, a 50% increase in digestive system deaths, and a 70% increase in deaths from other causes. Another major finding of the study was that no relationship existed between elevated cholesterol levels and cardiovascular deaths in women. In other words, the results of cardiovascular research in men simply do not apply to women!

My fear is that the public is being asked to accept long term treatment with diet and cholesterol-lowering agents when, in the final analysis, the treatment is more dangerous than the disease. This problem becomes even more important when our children become involved. I see little concern for the long-term harmful effects on growing bodies and brains when essential food substances are reduced or eliminated. In the final analysis, all we can say now is that some relationship exists between the level of cholesterol in the blood and the risk of a heart attack. However, that relationship is too weak to predict an increased likelihood of a heart attack in any given person. Certainly, there is no justification for mass screening of the general population for blood cholesterol levels. Nor is there reason for frightening patients into believing that if they lower their cholesterol, they will be less likely to have a heart attack. This is like believing that one can improve the weather by banging on a barometer.

Analyses of the plaques that line the walls of the coronary arteries have shown that only 5% of the plaques is cholesterol. [14] Accordingly, the belief that dietary fat and cholesterol cause coronary disease is just a myth, and its perpetuation is a huge scientific hoax. Unfortunately, this belief often obscures honest attempts to find the true causes and leads millions of people into changing their diets or taking drugs they don't need that have dangerous side effects.

REFERENCES

1. Ahrens, E.H. Dietary fats and coronary heart disease: unfinished business. *Lancet*, Dec. 22, 1979; 1345-1348.

2. McCormick, J. and I. P. Coronary heart diseases not preventable by dietary interventions. *Lancet*, Oct. 8, 1988; 839-841.

3. Lipid Research Clinic's Program. The Lipid Research Clinic's Primary Coronary Primary Prevention Trial Results. I. Reduction in the incidence of coronary heart disease. *JAMA*, 1984; 251: 351-364.

4. Lipid Research Clinic's Program. The Lipid Research Clinic's Primary Coronary Primary Prevention Trial Results. II. The relationship of reduction in incidence of coronary heart disease to cholesterol lowering. *JAMA*, 1984; 251: 365-374.

5. McMichael, J. Fats and atheroma: An inquest. *Brit Med J*, 1979; 278: 173-175.

6. Secondary Prevention in Survivors of a Myocardial Infarction. Joint Recommendations by the International Society and Federation of Cardiology Scientific Councils on Arteriosclerosis, Epidemiology, Prevention and Rehabilitation. *Brit Med J*, 1981; 282: 894-896.

7. May, G.S. et al. Secondary prevention after myocardial infarction: A review of long term trials. *Prog in Cardiovasc Disease*, 1982; 24: 331-362.

8. Oliver, M.F. Prevention of heart disease—propaganda, promises, problems, and prospects. *Circulation*, 1986; 73: 1-9.

9. Vitale, J.D., Ross, N. Critique of NIH Report on Lipid Research. *Consultant*, March 15, 1985, 141-150.

10. The Lipid Research Clinic– 83 –'s Program: The coronary primary prevention trial: Design and implementation. *J Chronic Diseases*, 1979; 32: 609-631.

11. Blankenhorn, D.H. et al. Beneficial effects of combined colestipol-niacin therapy on coronary atherosclerosis and coronary venous bypass grafts. *JAMA*, 1987; 256: 3233-3240.

12. Frick, M.H., Elo, O., Haapa, K., et al. Helsinki Heart Study: Primary-prevention trial with gemfibrozil in middle-aged men with dyslipidemia. *New Eng J Med*, 1987; 317: 1237-1245.

13.Jacobs, D., Blackburn, H., Higgins, M. et al. Report of the Conference on Low Blood Cholesterol: Mortality associations. *Circulation*, 1992; 86: 1046-1060.

14.Roberts, W.C., Kragel, A. H., Gertz, S.D., Roberts, C.S. Coronary arteres in unstable angina pectoris, acute myocardial infarction, and sudden cardiac death. *Amer Heart J*, 1994; 127: 1588-93.

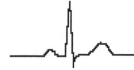

6.

THE DOCTOR-TECHNICIAN AND THE ANGIOGRAM

The test that has become a religion,
or, how to have unnecessary bypass surgery.

MOST YOUNG CARDIOLOGISTS elect to enter the field of invasive, or as it is now called, interventional cardiology. There are many reasons for such a decision but most invasive cardiologists have selected their field because they like to put catheters in hearts, do coronary angiograms, insert pacemakers, assist at cardiac surgery, etc. In some ways they are like people who climb mountains—they like to do it because it is there. In short, they have a built in bias to treat heart patients by doing something rather than by simply giving drugs. To put it succinctly, they are surgical cardiologists rather than medical cardiologists.

HOW TRAINING BIAS INFLUENCES THE CARDIOLOGIST

This bias towards active intervention profoundly influences the training of the young cardiologist, and the subspecialty he selects. While all future heart specialists are exposed in their training to the entire field of cardiology, that field has become so large that one person no longer can be expert in all its subspecialties. We now have general cardiologists, noninvasive cardiologists, pediatric cardiologists, nuclear cardiologists, echocardiographer cardiologists, research cardiologists, angiographer cardiologists, etc. Each one of these specialists spends most of his time in his own narrow specialty. Consequently, he becomes increasingly unfamiliar with the latest advancements in other areas. It is not surprising, therefore, that these doctors possess a limited view of how a patient with chest pain should be treated. Indeed, it would not be inappropriate to refer to these super specialists as technician-doctors because many of them behave more like technicians than doctors.

The critical reader should deduce from the above that there must be a variety of ways to diagnosis heart disease. That is true. While a lengthy discussion of each of these special areas is beyond the scope of this book, an exception to this is the angiogram. Except for the chest x-ray, the electrocardiogram, and the stress test, the coronary angiogram is the oldest and most familiar of the diagnostic tests used by cardiologists. If you are at risk of heart disease, it is essential you have some knowledge of what the angiogram will and will not show. Someday that information may save your life or that of a family member.

THE CORONARY ANGIOGRAM

A coronary angiogram is a procedure in which a flexible catheter (a long plastic tube) is inserted into a femoral artery, the main artery in the upper thigh. The catheter is pushed up into the femoral artery until it reaches the aorta, the main artery in the abdomen and chest—the one that delivers blood to the entire body. The cardiologist continues to push the catheter up the aorta until it reaches the heart. At this point the catheter is manipulated until it enters one of the main coronary arteries on the surface of the heart. When it is firmly within the coronary artery, a dye solution is injected under pressure so that it can fill the entire arterial tree. The dye is opaque to x-rays; consequently, when an x-ray is taken, the coronary artery and all its branches will be seen. Normally these arteries show smooth walls. As the artery branches, it becomes smaller and smaller until it can no longer be seen. When an artery becomes narrowed due to the presence of coronary artery disease, it looks very much like a straw that has been squeezed in the middle. The cardiologist can see this on a screen and will then estimate what percentage of the artery is narrowed.

Well over one million coronary angiograms are done yearly. Without the angiogram, the 390,000 annual bypass surgeries and the 350,000 annual coronary angioplasties could not be performed. While cardiologists claim the angiogram is the gold standard on which the diagnosis of coronary artery disease must be made, considerable evidence suggests that such is far from the truth; indeed, the coronary angiogram may well be one of the most inaccurate and misleading tests in the field of cardiology. Nevertheless, the economic rewards, as well as other motivating influences, appear to have distorted opinions of the true worth of this procedure. We'll discuss the economic factors in later chapters. Economics aside, many cardiologists have a religious like faith in the ability and accuracy of the angiogram to provide them with the guidance they need to treat their patients with chest pain. In fact, some are unable to function without its use.

HISTORY OF THE ANGIOGRAM

How reliable is the angiogram, and what is the evidence of its effectiveness? The angiogram was first introduced into clinical medicine by Dr. Mason Sones at the Cleveland Clinic in 1958. For the first time, the coronary arteries on the surface of the heart could be outlined and seen in the living patient. It was believed that narrowing of the coronary arteries would lead to chest pain due to coronary artery disease. The theory was that this narrowing would cause a proportionate reduction in the blood flow to the heart muscle, i.e., the greater the degree of narrowing of the coronary arteries, the greater the reduction in blood flow. Also, doctors thought that if the artery were completely obstructed, the heart muscle nourished by that artery received no blood. From these assumptions, it was easy to theorize that if the obstructed artery were bypassed, then blood flow in the artery would be restored and the heart would perform better. Patients with a significant narrowing of greater than 75% were thought to be at considerable risk of a heart attack. Those with severe narrowing, 90% or more, were felt to be in imminent danger of a heart attack in the very near future. Conversely, those patients in whom the coronary arteries were only mildly narrowed, by less than 25%, were considered to be in no danger.

The doctors of that time assumed the angiogram could tell them the cause of a patient's chest pain, whether the patient was at risk of a heart attack, whether or not he should undergo coronary artery bypass surgery, how he would respond to surgery, and what his ultimate prognosis was. Some cardiologists even went so far as to tell a patient he would die unless bypass surgery was immediately performed!

ASSUMPTIONS ON WHICH THE ANGIOGRAM WERE BASED DID NOT CORRELATE WITH CLINICAL PICTURE

All these assumptions were quite reasonable. However, after decades of study on tens of thousands of patients, these beliefs were found to be incorrect. One of the first discrepancies to become evident was the surprising fact that the severity of a patient's coronary artery disease did not correlate with his symptoms. For instance, advanced coronary artery disease, as shown on the angiogram, could exist in the complete absence of chest pain. Conversely, most patients with chest pain did not show the critical narrowing of a major coronary artery. Indeed, 10% to 15% of men and as many as 40% of women who complained of chest pain displayed normal or nearly normal coronary arteries. What was causing their chest pain?

Additional studies reinforced the belief that the information obtained from an angiogram repeatedly did not correlate with the clinical picture. Often an artery was found to be totally obstructed in a patient who had never had a heart attack or chest pain; instead the heart muscle supplied by that artery continued to function in a perfectly normal manner. Conversely, in other patients with impaired contraction, regular blood flow did not return to normal when the obstructed artery was bypassed, nor was the contraction of the heart muscle restored to normal.

Another misconception recently uncovered was the idea that critically narrowed arteries are in imminent danger of closing off and causing a heart attack. In one research project, patients were selected in whom two coronary arteries were found to be narrowed—one mildly and one severely. The patients were followed until they had a heart attack. At that time the angiograms were repeated. In the majority of cases, the artery with the most severe narrowing was not the one that caused the heart attack.

Similarly, in another study, patients were followed over a period of several years with repeated angiograms. Their symptoms were related to the progress of their underlying coronary artery disease. A poor correlation was found. For example, some patients would show a progression of their disease but still experience no change in their symptoms. Conversely, some patients had an increase in the amount of their chest pain, but their coronary artery disease appeared stable on the angiograms.

These latter observations should not have been a surprise. Autopsies have revealed for years that some people have severe coronary artery disease and yet their medical records showed no history of symptoms. In some cases an artery would be completely closed off. Yet, there was no history of a heart attack. Additionally, the well known Framingham Study established that as many as 25% to 35% of people showed evidence of heart attack on their electrocardiograms with the complete absence of symptoms. These are popularly called silent heart attacks.

Autopsy studies provided other valuable hints that the coronary angiogram was less than accurate in defining the presence or absence of coronary artery disease. Attempts were made to correlate the amount of coronary artery disease found on angiograms with the amount of coronary artery disease found at autopsy. Such studies invariably revealed a gross under estimation of the severity of disease as displayed by the angiogram. Commonly, patients thought to have only mild disease during life were found to have severe disease when studied after death.

Provocative findings came from attempts to determine if the amount of coronary artery disease found by one cardiologist would correlate with the amount of disease found on the very same angiogram by another cardiologist. Often the results were widely divergent. Cardiologist A might say the left anterior descending artery (the artery on the front surface of the heart) was only 40% narrowed, while cardiologist B would say it was 75% narrowed. Even when the same cardiologist read the angiogram at two different times without knowing it was the same record, the results often disagreed significantly.

Not only do angiograms provide inaccurate information, rarely do patients have more than one. Coronary artery disease takes place over many decades and there is no way a single angiogram can measure the rate of progress. To use a simple analogy, if I throw a ball up in the air, take a picture, give you the picture, and ask if the ball is going up or down, the answer will be, "I can't tell without another picture." In other words, it is impossible to tell whether the amount of narrowing has recently become worse, is no different, or is even improved over what it was five to ten years ago. Only serial angiograms can provide that information over time, and even then any disease progression may not correlate with symptoms.

Another major weakness of the angiogram is its inability to accurately determine the cause of a patient's symptoms. It originally was assumed that when a patient was having pain, the cause of that pain was narrowing of a coronary artery. From the studies already cited, it is clear that this is often not the case. Consequently, if we were to take the angiograms from 200 patients with coronary artery disease, only half of whom were having chest pain, and ask any cardiologist to tell us who they are, he will not be able to. An angiogram has no distinguishing features that can tell us which patient has pain and which patient is symptom free.

These inconsistencies cast doubt as to the credibility of the angiogram as a effective diagnostic test. Clinical experience and scientific studies have shown that an angiogram cannot determine the cause of a patient's chest pain. It cannot establish whether any coronary artery disease present is responsible for the patient's symptoms, or is merely coincidental. If coincidental, then perhaps there is another cause for the patient's chest pain. It cannot tell us whether the blood flow to the heart muscle is reduced, or whether it will be restored after bypass surgery. It cannot reliably tell us about the most important predictor of survival, that is, the function of a patient's heart, nor can an angiogram predict which artery will close off. Accordingly, it cannot predetermine if a patient is going to have a heart attack, or even whether his disease has recently become worse. It is unreliable in estimating prognosis, since the heart will ultimately develop its own bypasses, and it cannot forecast the response of a patient to bypass surgery.

MOST ANGIOGRAMS ARE UNNECESSARY

Why, then, is it necessary to have an angiogram, particularly if your symptoms are quite recent and no attempt has been made to control those symptoms with medication? Scientifically speaking, 95% of the time it is not necessary—all the information that an angiogram might provide, if it were accurate, can be obtained by safer, less expensive, and frequently, more informative noninvasive tests.

Unfortunately, most of the technician-doctors who like to do angiograms tend to disregard the information provided by noninvasive tests. Indeed, they also ignore the many limitations of the angiogram itself. In spite of its shortcomings they prefer to be guided almost solely by what they see on the angiogram. Sadly, they lack the basic knowledge to interpret what they see correctly and the result is an illusion.

It is essential that you understand the angiogram is the most over-rated test in clinical cardiology today. It is enormously over used; it makes more dollars than sense, and leads directly to unnecessary angioplasty or coronary artery bypass surgery. When should angiograms be performed? Not until the patient has had a maximum trial of medical therapy. As we shall see in later chapters, better than 90% to 95% of all symptomatic patients get better with the help of proper medication in adequate doses. Some even improve without medication. Only those who do not respond should undergo angiograms, for they may benefit from angioplasty or surgery. Yet some do not, and we can't predict who they may be.

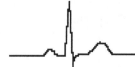

7.

CORONARY ARTERY ANGIOPLASTY

A new form of treatment,
or, the latest in medical experimentation?

All progress is made by dissatisfied people. Were it not for the pioneers in medicine, how we diagnose and treat disease today would be much as it was 50 years ago. Yet, that progress is achieved at a price. Rarely is the road to success a straight line. It abounds with wrong pathways and dead ends and, sometimes, dead patients. Also, no longer is a goal sought by a single medical scientist who finally reaches his destination through years of experience and failures. In our modern world with instant communication and shared knowledge, the researchers working on a problem may be numbered in the dozens or hundreds. While this speeds up acquisition of knowledge, and usually shortens the time to solution of a problem, it also increases the number of patients exposed to a new treatment along with its failures and complications. Human nature being what it is, successes are usually reported immediately while failures tend to be pushed into the background. At the same time, with many doctors and medical centers working with a new way to manage a disease, the public and doctors alike may mistakenly believe that the research is the new standard of care. The ultimate outcome may be one in which the new "treatment" may be more dangerous than the disease in some patients, but that information may not be recognized until it is too late for many.

CASE HISTORY

Susan Turner was thirty-eight, a mother of two children, ages eight and ten, the successful owner of an advertising agency. She had always been in good health but had little time for exercise or socialization. Her husband had not been as successful. He was a salesman, but because of the economy, his income was considerably less. This was often a source of friction, so much so that she now had to keep credit cards and charge accounts hidden and have the bills sent to her office. She didn't need this stress. Having to run a family, an ad agency, and cope with living was almost more than she could handle. The advertising business was stressful, customers were demanding and deadlines were tight. With her husband making so little money, she could not afford to lose even a single account.

While having lunch with a prospective customer one day she casually mentioned she wished she could handle the stress better. The customer volunteered that she worked out regularly at a nearby exercise center to get rid of her stress. This sounded like a good idea to Susan, besides, she needed to lose some weight. A few days later she filled out an application. Quite properly, she was informed that for the protection of both the customer and the exercise center, she would need a cardiac examination including a stress test. That seemed reasonable enough, particularly in view of the fact that her father had a heart attack when he was only 45-years old.

Susan called one of her friends, a nurse, to find the name of a cardiologist. Her friend recommended a local cardiologist whom she knew from the hospital. Susan was informed that he must be good because he always seemed to have patients there. She made an appointment for an examination the following week. He was very pleasant, asked her a few questions about symptoms, whether she smoked, did she still have her uterus and ovaries, was there a family history, and how stressful was her life. She confessed that she smoked about one pack per day, but she had no coronary symptoms. Yes, she had a hysterectomy after her last child because of excess bleeding; however, she was taking estrogens. After the preliminary examination and an electrocardiogram, a stress test was carried out.

To her surprise, the results of the test were abnormal. The cardiologist explained that whereas women, as a rule, didn't develop heart disease until after menopause, it was now more common to see younger women with heart disease because many were working and raising families at the same time. This could be very stressful. If, in addition, a woman smoked, had a family history, or had her uterus removed, she was at considerable risk of having coronary artery disease at a relatively early age. All four risk factors were true in Susan's case. He explained further that he could not be sure whether the stress test turned out abnormally because she had coronary artery disease, or if it were a false positive test. He elaborated that a false positive test was one in which the test results were abnormal, but the patient turned out to have a normal angiogram. He did not know why false positive tests occurred except that they were far more common in women. In order to resolve the dilemma, and to allow her to get on with her exercise program, he recommended an angiogram. He described what an angiogram looked like, and that it was a routine x-ray of the coronary arteries. He said the risk was minimal. Susan did not ask nor did he volunteer any information as to what he would do if coronary artery disease were found.

The following week she entered the hospital for her test. The angiogram was successfully carried out. She could see on the video screen that one artery seemed to be narrowed for a short distance. The cardiologist confirmed that the left anterior coronary artery was 50% blocked. There was a new procedure for this kind of problem. It was called balloon angioplasty. As a matter of fact more than thirty medical centers throughout the country were now treating coronary artery disease in this way. She was informed there was a risk in doing this procedure; however, she was told that the artery might close off at any time, and she could have a massive heart attack or die.

Susan was frightened. She could not afford to become ill. Who would take care of the children? She had always done most of the work at home, her husband didn't help much. In fact, she was almost a single parent. Besides, who would run the agency. Without the agency the family simply wouldn't have enough money to live on. Having the cardiologist remove the obstruction seemed like the best way out. She told him to proceed. "First, he said, we will have to get a backup surgical team in the event we have a problem. It will take about an hour to make all the arrangements."

The hour passed quickly with the help of a sedative injection. The next thing she knew the doctor was at work on her heart again. He explained he was passing a special catheter down the artery, and when he was finished he expected the blockage to be minimal. Suddenly she experienced excruciating chest pain. She dimly perceived that the doctor had become very excited and was calling for another doctor. The pain became worse and now was spreading to her neck, jaw and left arm. She could not lie still. Within a few moments she felt the jab of a needle in her right arm and soon the pain began to ease. The cardiologist anxiously told her that a tear had developed in the artery, and it would be necessary to perform emergency bypass surgery. They were taking her to the operating room immediately.

Susan was barely conscious when they wheeled her into the operating room. She could feel the mask slipped over her face. It was the last thing she would ever experience. The surgeons heroically tried to repair the tear in the artery but within a few minutes cardiac arrest occurred. All attempts at resuscitation failed.

Did Susan need this new procedure? Did the doctor do anything wrong? Could she have been treated in another safer way?

BACKGROUND

Although coronary angiograms were first introduced in 1958, it was not until 1977 that a cardiologist by the name of Andreas Gruentzig in Switzerland made the first direct attempts to remove the obstruction seen on a coronary angiogram. The idea was not a new one. In 1964, Charles Dotter, a radiologist, was the first to attempt the removal of an obstruction within the femoral artery of the leg using various sized catheters. For reasons that are unclear, the idea never caught on. Gruentzig expanded on the concept and developed a unique catheter with an inflatable balloon near the end. After perfecting the catheter in dogs, he extended its use to patients in whom an angiogram had demonstrated a localized obstruction in a single artery. The balloon catheter was inserted into the coronary artery until it reached its most narrowed portion. At this point the balloon was inflated under considerable pressure. Gruentzig's hope was that the material making up the arteriosclerotic plaque, and which was responsible for the narrowing, would be compressed by the inflated balloon, thereby opening up the artery for the normal passage of blood.

Gruentzig's idea was an exciting one. It attracted considerable attention when he presented his first four patients at the annual American Heart Association meeting in Miami in 1977. Within two years nearly 200 more patients had been treated in a similar way. The procedure was called percutaneous transluminal coronary angioplasty. With PTCA, as it came to be called, the cardiologist could immediately determine if the coronary artery obstruction had been reduced by repeating the angiogram. However, what made angioplasty stunningly different was that the cardiologist no longer had to call upon a cardiac surgeon to do bypass surgery. By removing the blockage himself, the fees that the surgeon used to command would now go directly to him. The temptation proved irresistible.

FORMATION OF A NATIONAL REGISTRY

Not surprisingly, in 1979, the National Heart, Blood and Lung Institute proposed that a National Registry be established. Very quickly 34 major medical centers agreed to contribute cases. In addition to these centers, a large number of other private and community hospitals began developing programs for angioplasty in their own institutions. These hospitals were under no obligation to inform the National Registry of their successes or failures.

Nor did they have to publicize the complications that occurred, or how long and difficult it was to learn this procedure.

LACK OF PUBLIC SAFEGUARDS

The fact that most hospitals and doctors were not required to report the results of their angioplasty studies to the National Registry revealed a major flaw in our medical system. Safeguards exist to protect the public from the side effects of new drugs. For example, a new drug must undergo four different phases of development each of which is under close scrutiny by the FDA. Who is allowed to use the drug is carefully controlled. Only experienced clinical investigators familiar with the problems that might occur with a new drug are permitted to do such studies. It may take seven to ten years before the drug reaches the market. Even then, if the FDA sees the drug has too many side effects after it is released to the public, it is quickly withdrawn.

In contrast, new procedures, such as angioplasty, have no such safeguards. A practicing cardiologist is free to take a brief course in angioplasties, and then can subject as many patients as he wishes to the new treatment. As long as he is reasonably careful, and has no more complications than other cardiologists, he is not likely to attract censure. Most cardiologists are cautious, since there is a real possibility that stretching a coronary artery will cause a dissection. A dissection is a complication of angioplasty. When an artery is stretched, the inside lining of the artery may tear. Blood then enters the wall of the artery and causes its muscular layers to separate. As a result, the artery may rupture, or the lumen of the artery may collapse and block the passage of blood, resulting in a heart attack. Accordingly, whenever angioplasty is performed, a backup surgical team waits in case emergency bypass surgery is necessary. Of course, this is another added expense to be paid by the patient. If emergency surgery does have to be performed as the result of complications with angioplasty, the mortality rate is very high.

Although reasonable attempts were made by most cardiologists to learn the new technique, most insurance carriers would not reimburse the doctor for his services until at least seventy-five angioplasties had been performed. It is not hard to predict how cardiologists reacted—they simply performed as many angioplasties as they could on anyone with chest pain. Here again, one of the medical profession's flaws is exposed. While an investigational drug must demonstrate clinical efficacy before the FDA will allow its release, no such requirement exists for a new surgical technique. Thus, even though no one really knew the long term consequences of angioplasty, it was quickly accepted as a new treatment for obstructive coronary artery disease, without any proof that the treatment was either safe or effective.

ETHICAL ISSUES

The introduction of angioplasty caused the disappearance of some of the traditional checks and balances that take place when one physician refers a patient to another physician. Typically, if a cardiologist had a patient with chest pain that he diagnosed as due to obstructive coronary artery disease, he would refer the patient to a cardiac surgeon. The surgeon then reviewed the case and decided whether surgery could be carried out successfully. Such a decision was usually based on evidence of obstruction as well as whether the artery was healthy enough to benefit. It would not do any good to bypass an obstruction if the artery downstream from the obstruction were so diseased and so narrowed that blood could not get through to the heart muscle. Additionally, the surgeon considered whether the patient was healthy enough to withstand surgery. No surgeon would operate on a patient with a high risk of dying on the operating table. If the patient's disease were too advanced, or if other major illnesses were present, surgery was more likely to be harmful than beneficial.

Prior to the introduction of coronary angioplasty, the patient's fate was in the hands of two skilled specialists who decided among themselves what was best for the patient. However, that changed with the appearance of angioplasty. Since the cardiologist no longer referred every patient to the surgeon, he became judge, jury, and executioner. He made the diagnosis, performed an angiogram to confirm the diagnosis, and made a decision as to whether the patient should be treated medically, or with angioplasty. Since the rewards were great for doing an angiogram ($1,000-$2,000), and even greater for angioplasty ($5,000-$7,000), a tremendous incentive existed for the cardiologist to convince himself of the needs, and benefits of these procedures. Often the cardiologist's zeal for angioplasty was not limited by whether the patient had extensive disease of the coronary artery downstream from the point of obstruction. Nor was it always influenced by how sick the patient was, or whether he had other complicating illnesses. Angioplasty does not require anesthesia or opening the chest, therefore, it is much less of a risk than open heart surgery. Consequently, when contraindications to bypass surgery were present, angioplasty has often been seen as a viable alternative, by competent as well as incompetent cardiologists.

SKILL

The matter of skill is worth mentioning here. A cardiac surgeon spends a major portion of his training in learning how to perform bypass surgery. Obviously a certain amount of skill is involved in surgical techniques. Those who do not possess the talent and the manual dexterity either never select surgery as a field, or change specialties when they learn they are not qualified. Thus, if a surgeon consistently demonstrates poor techniques, or has a high number of such dangerous complications as postoperative heart attacks, heart failure or deaths, other doctors will stop referring patients.

On the other hand, a cardiologist is not required to possess the great technical skill of a surgeon. Nor are there formal requirements for learning the intricacies of angioplasty. If this translates into fewer successes and more complications, the cardiologist is not likely to stop referring patients to himself. Even if a disaster develops following angioplasty, the information rarely filters out to the public.

LACK OF RESTRICTIONS IN PERFORMING ANGIOPLASTIES

At the time of its introduction into clinical medicine there were no legal, ethical or even moral restrictions to angioplasties. Almost any cardiologist who knew how to perform angiograms could perform angioplasty with only minimal training, consequently the speed with which angioplasty expanded was extremely rapid. It made the spread of bypass surgery look slow in comparison. It took 25 years for coronary artery bypass surgery to reach 350,000 cases per year—without angioplasty as competition. Angioplasty accomplished the same thing in less than 15 years, even against competition from bypass surgery.

This growth led the public to believe that studies had been carried out to prove angioplasty was a highly effective technique providing significant relief to patients with chest pain. Patients also assumed angioplasty had few complications and guaranteed no return of symptoms as well as averting future heart attacks or premature deaths. As we shall see, not only were these assumptions incorrect, but the treatment was often worse than the disease.

COMPLICATIONS OF ANGIOPLASTY

The first report from the National Registry appeared in June, 1982[1]. Thirty-four medical centers reported on a total of 631 patients who underwent angioplasty. Most of the subjects had disease involving only one coronary artery; 117 of these individuals (18.5%) had complications from the procedure. Six patients (1%) died, 29 patients (4%) had heart attacks, and 40 patients (6%) had to undergo emergency bypass surgery. Another 5 patients died within 3 years after discharge from the hospital. Approximately 98% of the patients were still alive at the end of 3 years. Three of the deaths occurred in comparatively young women of 38, 48 and 49 years. During the follow-up period of one year, 79% of the patients reported improvement in their chest pain. This statistic recalls a study performed in Europe and described in the next chapter in which 77% of the patients treated with placebo therapy improved.

In 1988 an additional study of the complication rate in the National Registry was described[2]. Some improvement was shown in the incidence of death, heart attack or emergency bypass surgery. A subsequent study[3] clearly showed that the rate of complications was related to the age of the patients. Patients under the age of 65 had an incidence of death, heart attack or emergency bypass surgery of 7.5%. However between the ages of 65-74 these complications were noted in 13% of patients. Above the age of 75, 17% suffered such complications. In this latter group, nearly 9% of the patients died. Similar results were reported by the Mayo clinic in a study of 752 patients who underwent coronary angioplasty. Here the incidence of death, heart attack or emergency bypass surgery was 18%, 20% and 21% for ages 65-69, 70-74, and above 75 years of age.[4] Clearly, the older the patient, the greater the likelihood of some major complication from the procedure. In these groups, there was a greater danger from the treatment than from the disease.

Keep in mind that, by this time, the centers reporting their complication rates were major medical centers experienced in performing angioplasty and they were voluntarily participating in the Registry study. There is no way of knowing what the complication rate was with inexperienced cardiologists working in smaller hospitals.

Perhaps a better reflection of the mortality rate following coronary angioplasty can be gleaned from the National Medicare Experience Study. This study is more representative of a cross-section of all cardiologists doing this procedure rather than a reflection of the experience of one or two skilled individuals at a major medical center. This study[5], the largest of its kind, summarizes the results in 96,666 Medicare patients who had either angioplasty (25,423 patients) or bypass surgery (71,243 patients). The thirty days and one year mortality rates for angioplasty were 3.8%, and 8.2% respectively! In contrast, mortality rates for bypass surgery were 6% and 12% for thirty days and one year.

One other major complication of angioplasty should be mentioned. This is the Achilles heel of this treatment. That complication is widely known as restenosis and occurs when a section of a coronary artery that was treated with balloon angioplasty becomes narrowed or obstructed again. Restenosis occurs in about 40% of patients who have angioplasty, and is usually accompanied by a return of the patient's symptoms. As a rule, the restenosis happens within a six-month period and the reasons for it are not known. Not surprisingly, it is the subject of an enormous amount of research. In spite of such research, we have seen no success in reducing the frequency of restenosis since the introduction of angioplasty in 1977.

A number of studies have attempted to find out whether emergency angioplasty would be beneficial in patients while they are having a heart attack [6-8,14-18]. In almost every instance the mortality and other complications were considerably higher than when angioplasty was performed in patients who were not having a heart attack. Paradoxically, this has not stopped many cardiologists from performing this procedure during such an attack.

HOW SUCCESSFUL IS ANGIOPLASTY?

By this time you must be curious as to whether or not coronary angioplasty is successful in relieving the chest pain associated with coronary artery disease? Also, how does the survival of angioplasty treated patients compare with medically treated patients or with those treated with bypass surgery? Usually when a new treatment is presented to the public, the success of the new method is reported in glowing terms. The emphasis is always on how many lives were saved. Side effects tend to be down played. But when angioplasty was introduced, it represented a totally new approach to the treatment of obstructive coronary artery disease. The impediment to arterial blood flow was visible on an angiogram; when the blockage was diminished or removed, the dye could be seen entering the vessel downstream. One could immediately see the decrease in the obstruction. Cardiologists claimed "angiographic success" in over 90% of the patients treated based on their observations of the increased blood flow, not based on how the patients felt or on how well they did in the future. Naturally, relief of symptoms was expected to follow.

HOW DOES THE CARDIOLOGIST DECIDE
WHICH ARTERY NEEDS ANGIOPLASTY?

We have already discussed in the last chapter how there are no distinguishing features in an angiogram allowing a cardiologist to determine with any dependable accuracy whether the obstructed coronary artery was the cause of the patient's chest pain. Although an angiogram might demonstrate less obstruction after angioplasty, how can the cardiologist be certain if that particular narrowed vessel was the cause of the patient's symptoms, especially when two or even three vessels are narrowed? If only one coronary artery is obstructed, as in the group of patients originally studied by Andreas Gruentzig, the angioplasty decision might not be difficult. However, many patients with obstructions of only a single vessel never have symptoms. Also, the frequency of heart attacks or premature death in patients with disease of only one coronary artery is so low that angioplasty is likely to be more dangerous than the disease.

A major problem in determining the success of angioplasty in preventing heart attacks is the question of which coronary artery is in greatest danger of completely closing off within the near future. Cardiologists have always assumed this would be the artery with the greatest degree of narrowing. For example, an artery that was 90% narrowed was thought more likely to become completely blocked than an artery that was only 25% narrowed. That's a perfectly reasonable supposition. Like so many other things in medicine, decisions and treatments are often based upon a hypothesis that ultimately proves to be false. Consequently, it was a shock to learn that an artery that was 90% occluded was less likely to close off completely than one only 25% narrowed. Studies to demonstrate this were done in a rather ingenious way. Dr. William C. Little of Bowman Gray School of Medicine studied the coronary angiograms of 42 patients who had angiograms both before and shortly after a heart attack.[9] Twenty-nine of these patients had a newly occluded coronary artery. In only 10 cases (34%) did the occlusion occur in the artery that was most severely narrowed on the first angiogram. In 13 patients (31%), the site of an occlusion could not even be determined from the angiogram.

Other investigators have approached the problem in a different way by studying patients with unstable angina. Unstable angina is the term applied to patients with new onset of chest pain or those who have an increase in their pre-existing chest pain. It has been shown that people with unstable angina are more likely to suffer a heart attack in the near future than those whose pain is unchanged or those with silent coronary artery disease. Indeed, this is the threat that many cardiologists use to frighten patients with unstable angina into immediate angiograms, angioplasty or bypass surgery. Accordingly, it must have been a disappointment for these doctors to learn that in patients who had angiograms before and after the onset of symptoms, the artery thought to be responsible for the unstable angina was often not narrowed on the first angiogram.[10],[11]

Since a cardiologist cannot always identify, with reasonable certainty, which diseased artery is responsible for a patient's symptoms, nor can he predict which vessel is likely to close off and cause a heart attack, how can he be certain which vessel needs to have angioplasty? He can't. To be more blunt, since angioplasty is a surgical procedure, the standards of surgery should be applied to angioplasty. Simply put, if a surgical procedure is to be performed, the surgeon must know in advance on which structure or organ of the body he is to operate. There are rare exceptions to this rule. For example, if an accident victim has internal bleeding from an unknown source, the patient will die unless surgery is performed as soon as possible. Since angioplasty is not, or should not, be carried out as an emergency procedure, it does not qualify as an exception.

IS ANGIOPLASTY JUSTIFIED?

If one is going to treat a disease without knowing whether it will benefit the patient, it is perfectly acceptable to do so as long as the therapy imparts no threat to the patient. It is not acceptable to offer a life threatening treatment that may be more dangerous than the disease. How then can angioplasty be recommended?

Angioplasty may be justified if more people are saved than lost. What, then, is the risk of coronary artery disease progressing to a heart attack or death? This is a critical question. One way to find the answer to this all important enigma would be to study patients suitable for angioplasty but who received only medical treatment. Two such studies exist. Dr. Mark Hlatky from Duke University investigated patients who had coronary angiograms prior to 1981 when angioplasty first became generally available. He selected 110 patients who had chest pain thought to be due to obstruction of the proximal portion of the coronary artery. This is the main trunk of the artery before it starts to branch. These patients were followed for 5 years. Their average age was 50 years. Ninety-seven percent of the medically treated patients were still alive at the end of this time, and only 15% had a heart attack. Thus, the annual death rate was well under 1% and the annual heart attack rate was only 3%.[12] These results are very similar to the statistics found in patients with disease of one vessel treated by angioplasty. The authors emphasized that 77% of the medically treated patients improved by six months compared to 78% of angioplasty treated patients in the National Registry. Thus, according to the limited amount of information available, angioplasty seems no more effective than medical treatment. In older patients it is a different story. The reader will recall the results of the National Medicare Experience Study in which the thirty day and one year mortality rates for angioplasty were 3.8%, and 8.2%. This is considerably higher than the mortality in the Duke patients.

It is worth noting that 56 of these 110 patients studied at Duke University were advised to have bypass surgery within six months of the angiograms. Of the surgically treated patients, at the end of 5 years only 91% were alive whereas 97% of the medically treated patients were alive.

The second study dealing with this question originated in France[13]. It dealt with the 10 year survival rate of patients who would have been candidates for coronary angioplasty had the technique been available. Ninety-six patients were followed for

10 years. Fifty patients had bypass surgery within six months of their angiogram. At the end of 10 years 90% of the surgically treated patients and 91% of the medically treated patients were alive. Thus, the annual mortality for the medically treated patients was about 1% a year. The quality of life of these subjects was said to be good. It was clear that the survival of medically treated patients was excellent in patients who would have been candidates for angioplasty had the procedure been available. Keep in mind that the medical treatment available during the time of these studies was far from ideal.

COMPARISON OF ANGIOPLASTY AND MEDICAL TREATMENT

Now comes the ultimate question. How does the survival rate and heart attack rate of angioplasty patients compare with similarly diseased medically treated patients matched for age and other characteristics? Unfortunately, that question cannot be at answered at this time. Unlike the major studies comparing bypass surgery to medically treated patients, no such comparative study has ever been performed with coronary angioplasty. For over a dozen years angioplasty has been done on hundreds of thousands of patients each year and no one knows whether it is successful, whether it prolongs life or prevents heart attacks! Doctors are convinced that removing or reducing the obstruction clogging a coronary artery will relieve symptoms. They think, or at least hope, that it will protect patients from future heart attacks and premature death. That may be true, but as of this writing in mid-1994 we have no evidence—17 years after the first patient was treated with angioplasty.

WHO SHOULD UNDERGO ANGIOPLASTY?

Who should undergo this high tech form of therapy? Logically, it makes sense to use angioplasty only when chest pain is so intolerable that it interferes with daily living, and when a patient fails to respond to appropriate medical treatment. In my experience, such patients are exceedingly rare. I have seen only three such individuals in the past 15 years. Patients invariably respond to a proper medical program, provided the doctor knows what drugs to administer and their correct dosages. Unfortunately, many physicians do not know how to do this because of the narrowness of their training and experience.

ARE WE DOING TOO MANY
ANGIOPLASTIES? IF SO, WHY?

If the benefits of angioplasty are unknown, if its risks are so great, if 40% of angioplasty patients have restenosis within six months, and if the response of a patient's chest pain to medical treatment is so outstandingly successful, then why are there more than 350,000 such procedures performed each year? Most critics believe the angioplasty industry is fueled almost entirely by the enormous financial rewards of the procedure. Support for this view is strengthened by comparing the number of angioplasties in the United States with those in the United Kingdom, a country most like us in its people and in the practice of medicine. In the U.K. in 1991, the latest year for which figures are available, 174 coronary artery angioplasties were performed per one million population. In contrast, this country saw 1,300 angioplasties per one million population[19].

Sadly, we once again come back to a fundamental problem in the practice of medicine. A new treatment has been put into widespread use without proof of its benefits. The roadside of medical care is littered with discarded treatments that doctors were convinced would be beneficial—radical mastectomy, hysterectomy, tonsillectomy, etc. Yet when subjected to the rigorous testing of controlled clinical trials, the claims could not be substantiated. The public must always remember that when a doctor recommends a relatively new treatment, even if it is in widespread use, you must demand to know whether there is adequate proof of its efficacy and safety. You must also ask what alternative forms of treatment are available. Ethically and legally, doctors are obligated to provide you with this information. If you don't request this information, you may be subjected to the latest in medical experimentation rather than the latest in medical treatment. But it is too late to do anything for Susan and her loss to her family.

REFERENCES

1.Kent, K.M. et al. Percutaneous transluminal coronary angioplasty: Report from the registry of the National Heart, Lung, and Blood Institute. *Am J of Cardiol.*, 1982; 49: 2011-2020.

2.Holmes, D.R. et al. Comparison of complications during percutaneous transluminal coronary angioplasty from 1977 to 1981 and from 1985 to 1986. *JACC*, 1988; 12: 1149-55.

3.Chelae, S.F. et al. Results of percutaneous transluminal coronary angioplasty in patients greater than 65 years of age from 1985-1986 National Heart, Lung, and Blood Institute's coronary angioplasty registry. *Am J Cardiol*, 1990; 66: 1033-1037.

4.Thompson, R.C. et al. Percutaneous transluminal coronary angioplasty in the elderly: Early and long term results. *JACC*, 1991; 17: 1245-1250.

5.Hartz, A.G. et. al. Mortality after coronary angioplasty and coronary artery bypass surgery. Natl Medicare Experience. *Am J Cardiol*, 1992; 70: 179-185.

6.Holland, K.J. et al. Emergency percutaneous transluminal coronary angioplasty during acute myocardial infarction in patients more than 70 years of age. *Amer J Cardiol*, 1989; 63: 399-403.

7.Kahn, G.K. et al. Timing and mechanism of in-hospital late death after primary coronary angioplasty during acute myocardial infarction. *Amer J Cardiol*, 1990; 66: 1045-1048.

8.Eckman, M.H.Z .et al. Direct angioplasty for acute myocardial infarction. *Ann Int Med*, 1992; 117; 667-676.

9.Little, W.C. et al. Can coronary angiography predict the site of a subsequent myocardial infarction in patients with mild-to-moderate coronary artery disease? *Circulation*, 1988; 3: 9-18.

10.Ambrosia, G.A. et al. Angiographic progression of coronary artery disease and the development of myocardial infarction. *JACC*, 1988; 12: 56-62.

11.Moise, A. et al. Unstable angina and progression of coronary atherosclerosis. *N Engl J Med*, 1983; 309: 685-690.

12.Hlatky, M.A. et al. Natural history of patients with single-vessel disease suitable for percutaneous transluminal coronary angioplasty. *Am J Cardiol*, 1983; 52: 225-229.

13.Danchin, N. et al. Ten year follow up of patients with single vessel coronary artery disease that was suitable for percutaneous transluminal coronary angioplasty. *Br Heart J*, 1988; 59: 275-279.

14.Ellis, S.G. et al. Randomized trial of late elective angioplasty versus conservative management for patients with residual stenoses after thrombolytic treatment of myocardial infarction. *Circulation*, 1992; 86: 1400-1406.

15.Simoons, M.L., Arnold, A.E.R., Betrie, A. et al. Thrombolysis with tissue plasminogen activator in acute myocardial infarction: No additional benefit from immediate percutaneous coronary angioplasty. *Lancet*,1988; 1: 197-203.

16.The TIMI Research Group. Immediate vs. delayed catheterization and angioplasty following thrombolytic therapy for acute myocardial infarction. TIMI IIA results. *JAMA*, 1988; 260: 2849-2858.

17. The TIMI Study Group. Comparison of invasive and conservative strategies after treatment with tissue plasminogen activator in acute myocardial infarction: Results of the Thrombolysis in Myocardial Infarction (TIMI) Phase II Trial. *N Engl J Med*, 1989; 320: 618-627.

18.De Bono, D.P. SWIFT trial of delayed elective intervention v. conservative treatment after thrombolysis with anistreplase in acute myocardial infarction. *Br Med J*, 1991; 302: 505-560.

19.Hubner, P.J.B. Cardiac interventional procedure in the United Kingdom during 1991. *Brit Heart J*, 1993; 70: 201-203.

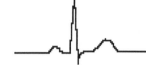

8.

HEART DISEASE

You may have only a mild case
but your doctor wants to operate.

A S A PRACTICING cardiologist who sees patients on a daily basis, I frequently hear stories from my patients about their friends, neighbors or family members who suddenly had to undergo coronary artery bypass surgery. Over the years I have heard these stories hundreds of times, and they all have the same scenario. It goes like this. "I just saw Joe a few days ago. He was working out in his yard and he seemed to be OK. We usually talk a couple of times a week and I had no idea he had a heart problem. Then he went to see a doctor because he had been having some chest pain. They operated upon him the next day!" Further inquiry usually reveals that the neighbor was told he needed surgery, not asked whether he wished to have it. Almost never do I hear that medication was tried for months, but failed to relieve the symptoms, and then bypass surgery was eventually recommended. Often I get a follow up report from my patient telling me his acquaintance had to go back for a second operation, or died. The sad thing about these scenarios is that a controversial form of treatment which came into being over 25 years ago, and which actually may be obsolete now, is presented to the patient with chest pain as the preferred treatment. Read on for a typical and true case history.

Tom Smith was 55-years old, happily married, and the father of two daughters. Lately, he had been noticing chest pain while working in his yard. Fortunately, in his job as a computer supervisor, he rarely had any strenuous exertion. Nevertheless, at other times that same squeezing pain would occur when he was working under stress. Usually, the pains disappeared within a few minutes. Tom was not too concerned and thought he had strained some muscles or was out of shape. His wife, however, noted he seemed more tired in the evening. Why didn't he see a heart specialist?

More to relieve his wife's anxiety than anything else, Tom decided to consult a cardiologist. The doctor briefly inquired about his symptoms, listened to his heart for a few moments, and then took an electrocardiogram. Next, Tom underwent a treadmill stress test but was unable to complete it because of chest pain. The doctor advised him he would "need an angiogram right away," and explained this was a "routine x-ray" of the coronary arteries on the surface of the heart. The doctor mentioned that it was his practice to do this test on all patients with chest pains. He was further told that he would be in the hospital just overnight.

Having no one else to advise him, and concerned about the results of the stress test, he entered the hospital for the angiogram. He was greatly impressed by all the high technology equipment. During the procedure he became the center of attention; doctors, nurses, technicians, and laboratory personnel all directed their efforts toward him. He had never seen anything like this before, except perhaps on television. A long, thin, plastic catheter was inserted into the main artery of his right leg, passed upwards into the main artery in the abdomen and chest and finally manipulated into one of the coronary arteries on the surface of the heart. Once in the artery, a dye solution was injected to visualize the artery on x-ray film. There was an intense feeling of heat throughout his chest followed by nausea and a desire to cough. Several more injections of dye were required before the procedure was finally completed. Each was accompanied by the warmth, nausea and cough. Finally, a large pressure dressing was placed over the thigh at the site of the catheter insertion, and he was told not to move his leg. At frequent intervals a nurse came in to check the pulse in his feet and look at the dressing. When Tom asked the nurse why this was being done, he was informed it was "routine." No one told him that there may be bleeding where the needle was inserted into the artery, or that occasionally the artery would become obstructed by a clot.

A few hours later, Tom's doctor approached his bedside accompanied by another physician dressed in a green surgical suit—a cardiac surgeon. They both had been reviewing his angiogram. Tom was gravely informed he needed a triple bypass immediately. He was led to believe that unless this operation was performed as soon as possible, he could have a massive heart attack and die!

Our poor patient was completely overwhelmed by all of this; he was thoroughly frightened and unable to think rationally. He was too intimidated to ask for another opinion; besides, didn't the cardiac surgeon review the films too? It did not occur to him to question his doctor and inquire whether alternative forms of therapy were available. He had heard there were many new and effective drugs for the treatment of coronary artery disease, but he assumed that in his case it must be too late for drugs.

Surgery was scheduled for the following morning. He was not allowed to have dinner that evening. An anesthesiologist stopped by and asked numerous questions about his health, his chest pains, whether he had any allergies to drugs, and if he had ever undergone surgery before. Tom was asked to sign an operative permit that he was too nervous to read. He was reassured it was just routine. His wife and both his children visited him and they were obviously worried. Well, he was too. What if he never survived the operation? The following morning while he was still asleep, he felt an injection in his arm. He tried to wake up but was groggy from the sleeping medication he had been given at bedtime. He was dimly aware as he was wheeled into the operating room.

Equipment, tubes, monitors and bright lights were everywhere. The anesthesiologist soothingly told him he was going to start an intravenous drip and to start counting to ten. It seemed he only got to three or four before he lost consciousness.

Tom had his surgery. Fortunately, it was an uncomplicated procedure that lasted about four hours. He awoke in the surgical intensive care unit with great pain in his chest and in the legs from which the vein grafts had been removed. He attempted to move his arms but they were both tied down. One had a clear solution dripping into his vein. The other seemed to be connected to some monitors along the side of his bed. He tried to talk but was unable as there seemed to be a tube in his throat. He found out later it was called an endotracheal tube; it was used by the anesthesiologist to administer anesthesia. Soon he realized there was one other tube entering his body. A catheter was in his penis, and it was very uncomfortable. Within minutes of his awakening a nurse leaned over his bed and asked him to nod his head if he needed medication to relieve his pain. He did so and within a short period of time gratefully went back to sleep.

At the end of the first day, the endotracheal tube was removed, but his throat was very sore, and he could barely talk. He continued to have a great deal of pain, which the pain injections relieved only in part. After 48-hours, he was transferred to another floor where one of the tubes was taken out of his arm. The catheter was removed from his penis as well. Unfortunately, he found himself unable to void, and it had to be reinserted for several days. Finally, all tubes and IVs were removed and he was allowed to gradually walk a little.

Eight days after entering the hospital he was discharged with a large scar down the center of his chest, and two long scars over both thighs. His legs were sore, his chest hurt, he was very weak, depressed, worried, and had two to three months of recovery to look forward to before he could return to work. In addition, he received a very large bill from the hospital ($28,000), a large bill from the heart surgeon ($10,000), and a third large bill from his cardiologist ($4,000). He also had smaller bills from the anesthesiologist, the surgeon who assisted the heart surgeon, and finally, one from the lung specialist whom he never remembered seeing in the recovery room because he was still unconscious. His total cost was over $42,000.

Slowly Tom recovered, but he continued to have sore legs and chest pain. The doctor reassured him these symptoms would eventually disappear. Most of them did except for a few twinges of pain in his chest now and then. Oh yes, he also had some residual swelling in one leg; it ached whenever he walked any distance. Tom had a temporary relapse after one month accompanied by chest pain, and rushed to see the cardiologist in the emergency room. He was informed one of the bypass grafts had closed off. However, "he had to expect these things, they happen." Little did he realize that closure of a graft meant that one of the bypasses had become occluded. The effect was exactly the same as if a major coronary artery had become obstructed. In short, closure of the bypass graft meant that the relapse and chest pain were actually symptoms of a heart attack, and he must have suffered some damage to his heart muscle.

Finally, he learned his insurance did not cover all his expenses, only 80% was allowed and he had to pay the difference, more than $8,500. Oh yes, he did receive an additional bill from the emergency room for $750.

Tom Smith's health and energy will be considerably poorer from now on. He began to talk about his problem to friends and relatives; he learned some patients had to undergo a repeat bypass after only three to five years. Only much later did he conclude, from reading, and talking to other patients and doctors, that his surgery was, in all probability, premature. Indeed, he could have been treated as safely medically, rather than surgically. He never had the benefit of other types of tests, particularly the noninvasive ones that often made angiograms unnecessary. Above all, no attempt was made for him take new and powerful drugs to relieve his symptoms. Ironically, the very heart attack he had hoped to avoid had occurred anyway, leaving him with permanent damage. What he did not know was that he had suffered additional damage to his heart from the surgery. This damage had nothing to do with the closure of the bypass graft, but was the direct result of injury to the heart muscle sustained during the operation. Had he not undergone surgery, but had merely suffered a heart attack, the damage would have been considerably less.

Tom talked to other patients with similar symptoms who had consulted less aggressive heart specialists. These patients were told that angiograms and bypass surgery were advised only when drug therapy had failed, and symptoms were persisting or becoming worse. Surgery was not a cure, only a quick fix. Apparently, these individuals had the benefit of more informed consent. They had been told that while surgery probably would relieve their chest pain, at the end of one year, many patients were no better, some were worse, and a substantial number were never able to return to work. Additionally, while surgery relieved symptoms, its benefits faded after only a few years in most patients.

Tom never asked, and therefore was never told, that his coronary artery disease must have been present for at least twenty to twenty-five years. The mere presence of the narrowing of a artery did not automatically mean it was going to close off. Nor was he knowledgeable enough to realize that a single angiogram, taken at just one moment in time, could not show whether his long standing disease had recently progressed, or was no different that it had been five or ten years ago.

Also, Tom was never informed that if he were treated medically with drugs, tiny new arteries, known as collateral blood vessels, would actually grow from nearby normal vessels to the obstructed artery, naturally bypassing the point of narrowing. Collaterals might also develop between segments of the same artery, from a point before the obstruction to a point beyond the obstruction. In effect, nature would create its own bypass. These collateral vessels would not transport the same volume of blood as the large arteries, but would be sufficient to prevent a heart attack. In fact, if Tom already had pre-existing collateral vessels, he may have lost them in bypass surgery.

No one had taken the time to explain to him that coronary artery disease can be turned into a benign illness by correct treatment. Wiser, poorer, disillusioned and depressed, Tom came to recognize the sad truth; there are far too many bypass procedures being performed, and most are probably unnecessary. Worst of all, he worried when his symptoms would return, and whether he would have to retire early. He could not afford that. Had the operation shortened his life?

9.

CORONARY ARTERY BYPASS SURGERY

Who needs it?
How often is it really necessary?

Some of the most incredible accomplishments of the medical profession have been in the field of cardiac surgery. Surgeons can repair defects in the muscular wall of the heart, replace or repair damaged valves, realign major arteries, cut out weakened sections of the heart muscle, and create detours for coronary arteries that are narrowed or obstructed. They can even replace a diseased heart with a new one. So essential are the contributions of the cardiac surgeons and their teams that it would be hard to imagine medicine without their help. Their skill in revolutionizing the field of cardiology in the second half of this century is one of the major accomplishments of our time.

Yet, the second half of the twentieth century may be remembered not for their monumental contributions, but for their unnecessary surgery on millions of patients for the misguided purpose of providing "new blood vessels" for those with coronary artery disease. Currently, nearly 400,000 people undergo coronary bypass surgery each year at an average cost of $40,000. Approximately $7,000 to $10,000 of this goes to the surgeon, $3,000 to $4,000 is paid to the cardiologist, and the remainder goes to the hospital. As we shall see, the majority of these surgeries are not only a wasted effort, but may materially accelerate the disability caused by the disease, and shorten the life span of those in whom the disease is relatively benign. After all, while 50% of the population die of cardiovascular disorders, 50% do not—many will live their normal life span and die of old age, or another disease—unless they have bypass surgery first.

Although bypass surgery provides temporary relief to the pain most patients experience from coronary artery disease, it comes at a very high price. Only about 25% of the subjects who have surgery truly benefit by receiving relief of their symptoms and a prolonged life. Unfortunately, it is not possible to predict in advance which patients will be included in that lucky 25%. Moreover, when the complications of this surgery are factored in, the treatment may be more dangerous than the disease for the remaining 75%. For example, of the 400,000 who have surgery each year, as well as the one million patients who have angiograms to find the surgical candidates, approximately 23,000 will die before discharge from the hospital, 25,000 will have heart attacks during or after surgery, 10,000 will have major strokes, 20,000 will have minor strokes, and 50,000 will have permanent cognitive defects with some loss of memory and reasoning after surgery. An additional 60,000 will obtain no durable pain relief from surgery. These numbers are conservative estimates, and do not include another 20,000 who have delayed complications anywhere from a few months to a few years after their operation. These include premature death, heart attacks, heart failure, and a host of other complications.

Thus, over 200,000 patients are worse after bypass surgery, versus the 100,000 who might benefit. The cost of this colossal effort is over twenty billion dollars a year! Sadly, most of these victims could have been successfully treated with medication at a fraction of the cost, and with little loss of life (1.5% to 2.0% per year), and few occurrences of a heart attack (2.0% a year). If those 400,000 patients were all on a reasonably good medical program, approximately 8,000 would have a heart attack and another 8,000 would die. Ironically, we have good reason to believe that the pain relief obtained at such tremendous cost is not solely from the surgical introduction of a bypass, but is coincidental to surgery—that is, other mechanisms are responsible for the disappearance of the patient's symptoms.

HOW BYPASS SURGERY BECAME FASHIONABLE

Coronary artery bypass surgery was first introduced in 1967 at the respected Cleveland Clinic as a major new treatment for coronary artery disease[1]. Dr. Rene Favalaro isolated and removed a long section of a vein from the inner aspect of a patient's thigh. Then he boldly isolated an obstructed coronary artery on the surface of the heart, and connected one end of the vein to a small hole that was created in the aorta a short distance from where it exited from the heart. The other end of the vein was sewn into the obstructed artery downstream from the obstruction. Now blood could flow directly from the aorta to the heart muscle, presumably helping the patient. At the time, there was little reason to question the need or the success of the operation. So enthusiastic was the response of the medical profession that by 1970 the Cleveland Clinic was doing 1,000 bypasses a year! For the first time here was a high technology treatment for the disease that was a product of our highly stressful civilization. Moreover, at that time, we had no long term effective medical treatment to either control the chest pain associated with coronary artery disease, or to prevent future heart attacks or premature deaths.

Few people failed to be impressed by the symptomatic relief of pain achieved by the operation. Never mind that the surgery was very expensive. After all it did require a high degree of skill and a great deal of very sophisticated equipment. The risk of dying and the complications of the procedure were acceptable, considering that coronary artery disease was thought to be a fatal disease at that time.

The operation and its apparent success captured the imagination of the American public and the world as no operation had ever done before. Generals, secretaries of state, movie stars, even kings had their bypass surgeries. Each time a public figure underwent such treatment, the media had a field day describing the spectacular results. Soon, almost by popular acclaim, bypass surgery became the standard of treatment for coronary artery disease. Patients with recent onset of chest pain, and who had never had chest pain before, were immediately admitted to the hospital and scheduled for angiograms. If coronary artery disease were found, the patient was not allowed to leave the hospital until bypass surgery was done. So eager were cardiologists and surgeons to operate, that repeatedly surgery was prescribed for patients whose only abnormality was a positive stress test. Indeed, one large hospital performed such surgeries on 500 patients who never had chest pain! Yet, in spite of all the hype, no scientific study had ever been completed that proved bypass surgery was as beneficial as it was claimed.

EFFECTIVENESS OF SURGERY BASED UPON TESTIMONY

Discordant facts emerged but were largely ignored by the medical profession and the public. One or two out of every ten individuals undergoing surgery did not get durable symptom relief, in spite of the fact that their obstructed arteries were bypassed. This meant that in these patients the coronary artery narrowing found on their angiogram was merely coincidental, and was not responsible for their chest pain. Therefore, there must have been another reason for their symptoms. In support of this possibility, case reports began to appear in the early seventies of patients with recurring chest pain who showed completely normal coronary arteries on angiography. Since their coronary arteries were not obstructed, was it possible for chest pain to have more than one cause? Ignored, too, were observations that some patients continued to have relief from symptoms even if their bypass grafts closed off after surgery. How could that be? Perhaps there was more than one mechanism, other than bypass surgery, whereby pain relief could be achieved.

Gradually other questions began to arise as to whether the bypass operation was successful in preventing heart attacks and premature death. Up until this time everyone had assumed the surgery was saving lives. No one doubted that it gave pain relief in most patients. But did it really protect patients from the complications of their disease? Would it prevent future heart attacks or premature deaths? Was it possible that some individuals were actually made worse by the surgery? Indeed, by this time, patients were coming back for a second operation, and some of them didn't do too well.

MAJOR SCIENTIFIC STUDIES FAIL TO SUPPORT EFFICACY OF SURGERY

Finally, in the mid seventies, three major scientific studies attempted to find out whether coronary artery bypass surgery was more effective than medical therapy. These studies looked at how successful surgery was in relieving symptoms, and how effective it was in preventing the complications of the disease. Two of these studies were carried out in the United States, and one in Europe, and involved 2,233 patients. These three studies found that while surgery was capable of relieving symptoms, it neither prevented heart attacks nor premature deaths. Indeed, at 10 years after surgery, a greater number of hospitalizations and heart attacks had occurred in the surgically treated patients than in the medically treated patients.

The first study to investigate the effectiveness of bypass surgery versus medical treatment was the European Coronary Surgery Study[2]. In this study, 767 patients were selected between the years 1973 and 1976. Medical treatment then consisted primarily of nitroglycerine-like drugs called nitrates. Isordil was the representative medication. A minority in this study received a relatively new type of drug known as beta blockers, of which Inderal was the prototype. These were the only medications available at that time. Such therapy today would be considered inadequate. After 5 years a survival advantage of surgery was found, 92% were still alive in the surgery group versus 84% in the medical group. The patients who had been the sickest received the greatest advantage from the surgery. Those with disease in all three coronary arteries and poor function of the heart showed the biggest benefits. However, for patients with disease of only one or two vessels and with good cardiac function, there was no significant difference in survival rates for those receiving medical versus surgical treatment. The study failed to show that bypass surgery protects patients from future heart attacks.

The second major study was the randomized Veterans Administration Cooperative Study[3]. This investigation compared the outcome in 686 patients who received either bypass surgery or medical treatment. This study also failed to find a difference in survival between surgically and medically treated patients. However, after 10 years, the cumulative heart attack rate was higher in the surgically treated patients (36%) than in the medically treated patients (31%). In part, this was due to the many postoperative heart attacks the surgery group suffered (13%), as well as in increase in heart attack rates after the fifth year (2.4% per year in the surgical group versus 1.4% per year in the medical group). The 10 year incidence of death or heart attack was also higher in the surgical group (54% versus 49%). Unfortunately, neither death nor heart attacks were prevented by surgery.[4]

The third and last major study was the Coronary Artery Surgical Study (CASS).[5] This was a fifteen-center study involving 780 patients, age 65 or less, with mild to moderate angina, and asymptomatic heart attack survivors selected from 1975-1979. One third had impaired cardiac function, 390 received surgery and 390 received medical treatment. Medical care consisted only of the beta blocker Inderal (in one-third of the patients) and nitroglycerine-like drugs. At the end of 5 years, the annual mortality in the surgically treated group was 1.1% versus 1.6% in the medical group. Patients with disease of all three coronary arteries, but normal heart function, had only a 1.1% annual mortality rate. The differences in mortality were not significant between the groups, i.e., bypass surgery saved no more lives than medical treatment. No difference was seen in rates of return to work, but the surgically treated patients did have more hospitalizations.

At the conclusion of these studies Dr. Eugene Braunwald, Chairman of the Department of Medicine at Harvard Medical School, summarized the results[6]. He stated that the effectiveness of coronary artery bypass surgery in relieving symptoms in 80% to 90% of patients was clear; therefore, chest pain that failed to respond to adequate medication was a legitimate indication for surgery. He noted, however, that most patients who undergo surgery are not resistant to medication; nevertheless, they receive surgery on the assumption that their chances of survival are better with surgery than with medical treatment. This assumption was not supported by three major scientific studies.

Dr. Braunwald also emphasized that considerable progress had been made in the drug treatment of coronary artery disease during the eight years it took to do these studies. As a result of advancements in medical therapy with beta blockers[7] (Inderal), aspirin[8], calcium channel blockers (Cardizem)[9], and the treatment of hypertension[10] the survival of patients with even more advanced forms of coronary artery disease had improved. He concluded that surgery should be reserved for patients whose symptoms were intolerable, and were not relieved by medical therapy, or for patients who were felt to be at very high risk on clinical evaluation.

A second editorial appeared two years later in *Circulation*, the official journal of the American Heart Association, by Drs. Thomas Kilip of Mount Sinai School of Medicine in New York, and Thomas J. Ryan of Boston University School of Medicine.[11] They made it clear that all three studies demonstrated that bypass surgery did not protect patients from a heart attack. Nor did it offer a survival advantage in those patients with good cardiac function. The only patients who appeared to benefit from surgery were those with a combination of severe coronary artery disease of all three vessels and poor cardiac function. Surgery also offered a survival advantage in those with disease of the left main coronary artery. Such disease occurs only in about 7% to 10% of the general population. Finally, they noted that the whole process of coronary artery obstruction speeded up by five to ten times in non-bypassed arteries. This meant that an artery that might close off in 20 years would now become completely obstructed in two to four years. The implication of the editorial was that surgery should be reserved for those who had disease of all three coronary arteries with poor cardiac function, and who responded inadequately to medication.

It is important to keep in mind that at the time of this research the medical treatment of coronary artery disease was extremely limited. Had these studies been done with modern drugs, medical treatment would have shown a clear advantage over surgical treatment, even in those with poor cardiac function. Thus, in spite of the popularity of bypass surgery, its unpredictable benefits may be limited to only the small minority of patients who fail to respond to appropriate medication. In the group who would be expected to respond equally well to surgical or medical treatment, surgery offers no survival advantage, and exposes the patient to the many complications of such surgery.

COMPLICATIONS OF BYPASS SURGERY

I cannot discuss the perceived benefits of coronary artery bypass surgery without mentioning the complications and side effects of this procedure. These tend to be glossed over when surgery is being discussed. It is doubtful that most patients who are urged to have surgery are really given enough information to make an informed consent. So you may be surprised by the number of complications that can occur.

The most important complication of surgery is, of course, the immediate as well as the delayed death rate from the operation. Surgeons have a natural tendency to minimize the mortality associated with the procedure. It is not uncommon to hear that the immediate mortality of such surgery is only 1% to 2%. That statistic may be true with a highly skilled surgeon and surgical team, and a relatively young patient with a good functioning heart. It is certainly not true for the average hospital in this country dealing with an older patient.

Several years ago the *Los Angeles Times* carried out the largest survey of its kind and studied the mortality associated with bypass surgery in nearly 17,000 patients in California.[25] The death rate ranged from 1.6% to almost 15%, with the average at about 5.5%.

Evidence shows that the same variation exists throughout the rest of the country. We would all like to think that well-known institutions are safe places to have heart surgery. Unfortunately, that is frequently not the case. For example, the 1987 mortality rates for bypass surgery on Medicare patients[26] (the only year for which national mortality data are available) reveals that at Henry Ford Hospital in Detroit, 89 bypass surgeries were done, at Grossmont Hospital in La Mesa, California, 68 surgeries were done, and at Missouri Baptist Hospital in St. Louis, 218 surgeries were done. The mortality at each of these hospitals was under 1%. In contrast, at the University of Chicago, 57 surgeries were performed with a mortality of 22.8%. At Parkland Hospital in Dallas, 32 surgeries were performed in 1987 with a mortality of 21.9%. At St. Joseph Hospital in Burbank, California, 70 surgeries were performed with a mortality of 20.0%.

Other factors affect the mortality of bypass patients, most notably the age of the person.. Only 1% of forty-year-olds might die as a result of bypass surgery, 3% of fifty-year-olds, 5% to 6% of those in their sixties, 7% to 8% in the seventies, but over 10% of the patients in their eighties. Mortality is greatly influenced by other diseases that might be present. For example, a 55 year old patient who has had one or two heart attacks, might be at greater risk than a 70 year old who has never had a heart attack, and has a normally contracting heart. Diseases such a emphysema, diabetes, kidney disease, hypertension, vascular disease elsewhere in the body can heavily influence mortality, as does the fact of whether the patient is a cigarette smoker.

In addition, the level of skill of the surgeon, the experience of his team, and the quality of the post operative care has an enormous impact on survival. Thus, a 65-year old patient with emphysema, diabetes and a prior heart attack may actually be safer in the hands of a highly skilled surgeon than a 45 year old with no prior heart attacks, but who is at the mercy of an incompetent cardiac surgeon.

Large medical institutions have marketing departments and advertise heavily. In 1988, hospitals spent $1.3 billion on marketing and advertising. It is their job to see that their hospital or medical center receives a lot of favorable publicity. The hospital may be well known because of the research they do. This is not a guarantee they have skilled surgeons. A few years ago, one of the large medical schools in this country was in the embarrassing situation of having its cardiology department refer potential surgical candidates to surgeons in other hospitals and cities. The mortality rate of the medical school surgeons was far beyond what was considered acceptable. The head of the cardiology department ultimately resigned rather than send patients to the medical school surgeon. It is absolutely essential when bypass surgery is considered, that the patient and family insist upon knowing the mortality rate of the surgeon who is operating, and not rely on a statistic from the medical literature.

The second major complication of bypass surgery that should be mentioned is a heart attack. Almost invariably after a patient has angiograms, a cardiologist will urge bypass surgery or angioplasty because a vessel is highly narrowed. The patient will be told the vessel could become completely obstructed at any time and cause a heart attack. I emphasized in previous chapters that it is not possible to foretell whether an artery will become completely obstructed unless it is already 98% to 99% closed. Nevertheless, cardiologists and surgeons frighten patients into having surgery, even when only moderate obstruction is present. On the other hand, they tend to ignore the probabilities of a heart attack *after* surgery. Not many studies have dealt with this subject because it is difficult to determine whether the changes in the heart muscle are due to a heart attack or to the surgery.

Surgery represents a form of injury to the heart muscle. When a surgeon operates on the heart, it must be handled, moved around, cut into, and dissected. When this happens, there are apt to be enzymes liberated into the blood stream from the damaged muscle, and changes in the electrocardiogram. A heart attack is also a form of injury to the heart muscle. It, too, will result in the release of enzymes into the blood stream and changes in the electrocardiogram. Indeed, this is how we make the diagnosis. Thus, it is hard to determine after surgery what is surgically-induced injury, and what might be a heart attack. Accordingly, the incidence of post operative heart attacks varies from only a few percent to as high as 20%, depending on the report being cited. In all probably the incidence is from 5% to 15%. Thus, it is not possible to predict whether a patient with a narrowed coronary artery is more likely to have a heart attack without surgery than with surgery. Anyone who claims he can make this prediction is either uninformed, or is misleading you.

There is one special type of injury to heart muscle that is so common after surgery that surgeons and cardiologists lightly consider it a normal post operative effect and constantly ignore it. I am referring to a change in the contraction pattern of the muscular ventricular septum that divides the heart into a right and left ventricle. Normally, the two walls of the heart approach each other during contraction and move in opposite directions as the heart fills with blood. At the same time the heart muscle thickens during contraction in the same way as the biceps muscle thickens when you flex your arm. After bypass surgery the ventricular septum will commonly lose both these functions permanently. This is quite serious and can severely compromise the function of a diseased heart.

The next most serious complication that occurs after bypass surgery is a stroke. Major strokes, such those leading to a complete loss of function of an arm and a leg and severe impairment of speech may be seen in 1% to 2% of patients undergoing surgery. The rate is considerably higher in patients in their seventies, and as high as 9% for patients in their eighties.[27] The frequency of minor strokes causing weakness of only one extremity or a slight impairment of speech is also high, perhaps as much as 5% to 10%.

Another type of complication that may occur in the brain is a loss of cognitive function. A study of 900 patients at nine medical centers in the US., Europe and South America found that 23% experienced impaired reasoning and memory loss after bypass surgery, according to Dr. Allen Willner of Hillside Hospital-Long Island Jewish Medical Center. About 10% of these patients will show improvement. Subtle personality changes are not at all uncommon but are very difficult to measure. Families will report that the recipient of surgery will show personality changes, or simply a loss of sharpness. Such symptoms probably go unrecognized by the patient's doctor, but are apparent to members of the family.

Of great interest is a study detailing the complications reported several years ago from one hospital in California after an analysis of 365 consecutive bypass patients.[28] Major events (such as a heart attack or death) were noted in 13% of the patients who had major complications. Major complications of bypass surgery included: hemorrhage into the chest cavity, rhythm disturbances requiring a pacemaker, hemorrhage in the space between the heart and pericardium, heart failure, pneumothorax (air in the chest cavity) requiring a chest tube, spontaneous opening of the chest incision, infection of the breastbone, heart attack, stroke, bacterial endocarditis (infection of the inside lining of the heart), aneurysm (ballooning out of a wall of the aorta), pulmonary emboli (clots in the lung originating from inside the heart), kidney failure, septicemia (blood poisoning), and cardiac arrest. A number of minor complications occurred, including thrombophlebitis (clots in the leg veins) and paralysis of one side of the diaphragm. Not mentioned in this study but possible were loss of cognitive function, loss of motion of the ventricular septum, increased progression of the patient's coronary artery disease, hepatitis and AIDS. While the reader may not fully understand many of the complications, the point is that the number that do occur, even in good hospitals, is substantial. Sadly, warnings about such complications are rarely made available to a prospective bypass candidate or his family.

In addition to these major side effects, other reports have indicated that about 15% of patients have minor side effects. Thus, between 25% and 30% of patients undergoing bypass surgery have either a major or minor complication.

One complication fails to be mentioned in most studies. A large proportion of bypass patients are unable to return to work. No doubt there are many reasons for this, as one may deduce from the number of adverse effects that may occur, but loss of one's job and inability to function have a devastating effect on the victims. The surgeon or cardiologist, however, no doubt would classify these poor souls as successful surgeries because they no longer have chest pain.

WHY PATIENTS WITH CHEST PAIN ARE RELIEVED BY BYPASS SURGERY

In spite of the numerous complications that accompany bypass surgery, many surgical cardiologists still advise it because it is effective in quickly relieving the symptoms of coronary artery disease in most patients. Unfortunately, such relief is often only temporary. Accordingly, it would be appropriate to review why patients who have bypass surgery do find some relief from their symptoms.

If you were to develop chest pain due to coronary artery disease and bypass surgery relieved your symptoms, no doubt you would assume that the elimination of your chest pain was the result of your obstructed arteries being bypassed. This rational assumption is almost a religious belief held by most surgeons and cardiologists, and that belief is passed on to their patients. However other explanations exist why patients find relief from their pain.

But let's step back a bit; to begin with, anywhere from 10% to 20% of bypass patients do not feel any pain relief. Why not? Another 10% have a return of their pain within twelve months, even though their grafts remain open. Why? An additional group of patients will have complete closure of all their bypass grafts and yet remain symptom free.[13,14] How can this be? Each of these observations suggests that coronary artery disease may not be the sole reason for chest pain , nor is the insertion of a bypass the only reason why such pain disappears after surgery.

One of the most powerful supports to this view is the dramatic effects of a placebo operation. In these strange studies, patients with recurring chest pain were taken to the operating room and anesthetized. Instead of a bypass operation, all they received was a skin incision. Each of these patients had improvement in their symptoms after this phony surgery.[15,16] Perhaps the attention and care convinced them they felt better even though the surgery couldn't have possibly improved their condition. The placebo effect is very powerful and rather mysterious, but it has been proven to exist in a myriad of different studies.

Another important reason to support the view that relief of symptoms is not dependent upon the bypassing of an obstructed coronary artery, may be found in patients who were operated on in the forties, fifties and early sixties before the technique of by-pass surgery was ever discovered.[17] In these operations, attempts were made to supply the heart muscle with new blood vessels in a variety of ways.[18] Some of these procedures were able to achieve pain relief in as many as 85% to 90% of the patients. Even today this would be considered good results.

Our intriguing question remains: why do most bypass patients obtain relief from their pain? Besides the placebo effects of the operation, there are several reasons why this spontaneous pain relief may take place. One is the circulatory system's ability to develop new vessels that grow from healthy arteries and attach themselves to the obstructed artery downstream from the obstructed segment. In this way the heart repairs itself and blood is able to flow around the blockage to supply the heart muscle. These new vessels are called collaterals and will be taken up in more complete detail with illustrations in a later chapter.

How effective are these healing processes of the heart? The vast majority of patients who develop angina will spontaneously improve even in the absence of any kind of treatment. One of the first reports to demonstrate this was from Ireland in 1981. Dr. Risteard Mulcahy at St. Vincent's Hospital in Dublin studied 101 patients with stable angina. [19] Patients between the ages of 35 and 74 were treated conservatively without any modern drug therapy. The 28 day mortality was only 4% and the 1 year mortality was 10%. Nine percent developed a heart attack within 28 days and 3 % more by the end of the year. These figures compare favorably with other treatment procedures.

Several other reports have appeared all dealing with the placebo treatment of patients with angina pectoris. [20-23] These show that angina patients can be treated quite safely with rest, avoidance of stress, and sublingual nitroglycerine to relieve the acute attacks. The heart attack rate and the mortality rate were quite low in these investigations compared to the mortality seen with surgical treatment. For example, in the recent study by Professor J.P. Boissel in France, 35 patients with at least five attacks of chest pain per week were studied for a period of six months. All were given placebo tablets daily. The only medication permitted was sublingual nitroglycerine for pain relief. At the end of this time, chest pain had diminished to an average of two incidents per week and 77% of the patients were considered significantly improved. During the period of the study, there were no heart attacks or deaths, and none of the patients needed to have bypass surgery.

Another powerful reason why patients experience pain relief from bypass surgery could be the weight loss that often accompanies it. There seems to be something about having one's heart operated upon that causes patients to lose their appetite. Many lose a great deal of weight. Loss of weight means a reduction in fluid retained by the body, and a significant decrease in workload for the heart. A reduction in weight is a cornerstone of all treatments for patients with chest pain, but is rarely achieved. Its net effect is equivalent to increasing the available blood to the heart muscle. In short, it is an effective treatment for patients with chest pain. No doubt it is also the reason why patients with chest pain obtain relief with low cholesterol and low fat diets. Such diets also happen to be low in calories and are associated with a significant reduction in weight in those people who adhere to it.

Another reason why people may get relief from angina after bypass surgery is the combined effect of bed rest and the absence of stress during the convalescent period. This period of rest and relaxation may last anywhere from one to three months and can have a profound influence on blood pressure. The effect of stress upon the heart was fully discussed in another chapter. However, it is not generally known, even by many cardiologists, that high blood pressure is a frequent cause of recurring chest pain.. Patients, even with a very high blood pressure, will have a fall of their pressure, often to normal levels, with bed rest. Whether it is bed rest alone or relief from the stress of daily living, there is no question the great drop in pressure occurs. Such marked reductions in pressure have multiple effects including a decrease in the workload on the heart, an increase in blood flow to the heart muscle, and a reduction in heart rate. It is not surprising, therefore, that bed rest is one of the most effective ways of obtaining pain relief. Unfortunately, it is not very practical when a patient has to work every day. However, since the recovery period following bypass surgery takes several months, the blood pressure not only stays down during this entire period but remains down for a long period of time afterwards—perhaps as long as six to 12 months. This may be the reason why many patients are pain free for several months, only to have a return of their symptoms within the next year. Obviously such patients do not need bypass surgery, they need blood pressure medication.

Still another reason for pain relief is the elimination of cigarette smoking. Many patients will finally quit smoking after bypass surgery. Presumably, the prolonged period in the hospital, the trauma of surgery, and the handicaps of the recovery period help break the habit. Everyone knows (or should know by now) that cigarette smoking is a major reason for the development of premature heart disease. Nicotine not only greatly accelerates the development of coronary artery narrowing, but also significantly reduces the oxygen carrying capacity of the blood. This occurs because the carbon monoxide produced by the cigarette has a greater affinity for the hemoglobin molecule than oxygen. In heavy smokers, even when they aren't smoking, as much as 20% of the oxygen carrying capacity of the red blood cell is taken up by carbon monoxide. All of us would like to receive a 20% increase in income. That's what the heart gets when cigarettes are stopped and the blood stream can finally carry its full load of oxygen.

Many patients with recurring chest pains are badly out of shape and haven't exercised for years. Exercise rehabilitation programs are a standard feature after bypass surgery in many parts of the country. Such programs are thought to encourage the growth of new vessels in the region of the narrowed coronary arteries, allowing the blood to detour around the obstructed vessels. To be sure, this is what the surgeons do with their bypass procedures. However, bypass grafts frequently close off or become narrowed again. The growth of the body's own collateral vessels is more permanent, and helps to provide blood to the heart muscle.

Still another reason why pain relief occurs after bypass surgery is that pain fibers going from the heart to the pain center in the brain may be cut during surgery. How often this occurs is difficult to say. This same mechanism is responsible for the absence of chest pain in patients who have had a cardiac transplant. It is common knowledge in the cardiology field that patients who receive a heart transplant will no longer experience chest pain, even though the transplanted heart develops severe coronary artery disease. One of the interesting side effects of cardiac transplantation is the development of severe coronary artery disease in the recipient. Indeed, other than rejection, accelerated coronary artery disease in a transplant recipient is the most common cause of death. Most transplant patients now have coronary angiograms annually to track the progress of their coronary artery disease. However, no matter how severe it is, the victim never has chest pain because all the pain fibers of the heart were severed when the heart was removed from the donor.

The next reason why bypass patients may feel pay relief is because a heart attack may take place during or after surgery. If you put a tourniquet around your arm and partially shut off the blood supply, it wouldn't take long for your arm to ache. This is because the body tissues produce lactic acid and other metabolic products that stimulate the nerve endings. Normally all of the body's waste products are constantly removed by the blood. When the blood supply to the heart muscle is reduced, then the rate of waste product removal also will be curtailed. When an individual with coronary artery disease is at rest, ordinarily he has no symptoms because the blood supply is adequate to remove any lactic acid and other metabolites from the heart. With exertion, the heart works harder and produces more waste products. Now the rate of removal cannot keep up with waste production and the patient feels pain. However, this process only occurs if there is living heart muscle to produce the metabolic byproducts. If a heart attack occurs during or after surgery, part of the heart muscle dies. This means it can no longer produce waste; with no waste there is no pain. Since heart attacks occur in 5% to 15% of patients having a bypass, these individuals won't have any pain, providing they survive.

A more subtle mechanism may account for some pain relief. The tough membrane that surrounds the heart (known as the pericardium) is cut open during surgery in order to access the heart, and it is left open after the patient's chest is closed. One of the changes that occurs when a patient develops chest pain is that the heart muscle temporarily becomes stiff, presumably because it becomes engorged with blood. This results in a loss of elasticity in the area where the blood supply is deficient. Since the muscle can no longer stretch and expand when the heart fills with blood, there is a rise in pressure within the heart's chambers, specifically, the left ventricle and left atrium. This increased pressure is transmitted equally in all directions. It is not unlike blowing air into a balloon causing it to expand. As long as the pericardium is intact, it limits the expansion of the left ventricle when it fills with blood. In the normal heart this is not a problem. In the diseased heart, since the expansion of the ventricle is limited, the heart muscle itself is compressed against the pericardium thereby increasing the pressure within the muscle. The effect would be similar to placing a raw steak between your hands and pressing your

hands together. The blood will be squeezed out of the steak because the blood vessels are being compressed. In the case of the
heart, the increase of pressure within the muscle compresses the
tiny blood vessels causing the blood flow to slow down or even
stop. When this happens the patient develops chest pain. After
surgery, since the pericardium is no longer intact, it cannot restrict the expansion of the left ventricle. Therefore, the pressure
within the chamber does not rise as it did before, even though
areas of the heart are still less elastic. Since the muscle is no longer
compressed, the small vessels within the muscle retain their normal size, blood flow is not reduced, and chest pain does not occur.

Whenever I give lectures on the subject of bypass surgery, and
even hint that sometimes it is not necessary, the most angry and
hostile questions come from those who have already had the procedure. Many of these patients swear by the surgery and claim to
be living pain-free now. Could this recovery be somehow associated with the huge cost of the surgery. When something costs
$40,000, the psychological investment has to be large too, and the
need to feel better is very strong.

HOW OFTEN IS BYPASS SURGERY NECESSARY?

It should be evident there are many reasons why patients obtain relief from their symptoms after bypass surgery that have
nothing to do with bypassing the obstructed coronary artery. In
spite of the strong probability that alternative mechanisms may
be responsible for relief of symptoms in many patients with coronary artery disease, thousands of physicians still recommend
surgery first and operate as quickly as possible. Thus, when the
surgeon says to the patient, "We weren't a moment too soon,"
what he really means is that if there were any further delay, the
patient might have recovered on his own. This brings up the question of how often is surgery really necessary?

A telling answer to this question comes from a study of 150
patients who were advise to have bypass surgery but refused.[24]
The subjects were followed for up to eight years. They did receive modern drug therapy. For those with disease of only one or

two coronary arteries, the annual mortality rate was 0%! For those with disease of all three vessels or the left main coronary artery, the annual mortality was only 1.3%—far below what the immediate surgical mortality would have been. Overall survival at eight years was estimated to be 89%. Other studies of patients who have refused surgery have shown similar findings.[12] Indeed, for those who refused surgery, the death rate after four years was lower than it was for those who chose surgery.[29]

In view of the many complications and side effects associated with bypass surgery, and particularly in light of the failure of major studies to document the effectiveness of surgery in either preventing heart attacks or premature deaths compared to medical treatment, why do cardiologists continue to recommend, and surgeons continue to carry out such surgery? Instead of decreasing, the number of surgeries for coronary artery disease has grown at an astonishing rate. This is particularly remarkable since balloon angioplasty is also widely used to open up the coronary arteries.

Part of the reason surgery continues to be preferred is because the cardiologist is heavily influenced by factors such as his own economic needs, his experience and ability to use medical treatment, his need for the prestige that angiograms and surgery offer, his need to do a certain number of angiograms each year to maintain his hospital privileges, whether he is employed by a hospital and is expected to keep the operating rooms full, and even whether the patient would be part of a research study and, therefore, is needed to fill a quota. In some instances the doctor may be concerned about a possible malpractice suit should surgery not be advised, and the patient has a heart attack or dies.

How, then, can anyone, public or doctors alike, decide how often bypass surgery is really necessary? They can't unless informed cardiologists speak out. In my opinion such surgery is rarely necessary. In my cardiology practice, only two patients have had bypass surgery in the past twelve years. All the remainder have been treated successfully with medication. Heart attacks, the need for hospitalization, and premature deaths are extremely rare in these individuals—far below the average seen in those who do have surgery. Other noninvasive cardiologists might disagree with my statistics a bit, but the important fact is that the great majority of people with coronary artery disease can be successfully treated with modern drug therapy without the need for an operation.

BYPASS SURGERY DURING AN ACUTE HEART ATTACK

There is one further clinical situation you should be warned about. Many cardiologists and hospitals have urged patients in the midst of a heart attack to have immediate bypass surgery or angioplasty. In this situation, the helpless patient may find himself in some strange emergency room in the middle of the night with a doctor he has never seen before. Usually he has had a sudden onset of crushing chest pain of great severity and was rushed to the nearest hospital with a suspected heart attack. We have little advance warning of this kind of catastrophe. The patient is in severe distress, is frightened for his life, is intimidated by all the medical personnel around him taking EKGs, x-rays, drawing blood, attaching monitoring electrodes, administering oxygen, and starting IVs. When the doctor in the white coat says "We must do emergency angioplasty or bypass surgery to save your heart," you're in no position to argue. Unfortunately, I think you must argue. We have no evidence that bypass surgery is more effective than medical treatment in this situation. Indeed, it may be more dangerous. Similarly, the majority of studies on emergency angioplasty for heart attacks have shown that the death rate is higher than with conservative medical treatment, except perhaps in rare cases when the patient is in shock due to a massive heart attack. Once again, this is not the latest in medical treatment, but the latest in medical experimentation.

In another scenario the cardiologist will recommend a routine angiogram for a heart attack patient before he leaves the hospital, even when his convalescent period has been uneventful and pain free. The cardiologist will claim that its purpose is to determine prognosis and to guide his treatment. The test is not without risk, and the information it may provide so shortly after a heart attack will be useless if the patient is without symptoms. Such an angiogram is not for the patient's benefit but for the cardiologist's benefit. If you are asked to undergo such a study before discharge, and you are not having any more chest pains, simply refuse.

Since ancient times, the medical profession has been guilty of adhering to old fashioned and obsolete forms of therapy. Coronary artery bypass surgery was introduced in the late sixties to help with the problem of chest pain due to heart disease, for which there was no effective therapy at that time. It remained a successful therapy for many years. Today, we have numerous drugs that will relieve these symptoms. Thus, there is rarely a need to adhere to older forms of treatment. Doctors who refuse to give up older procedures may be well meaning but misguided. A physician who has your best interests at heart should present you with all available options for treatment, along with their advantages, disadvantages and side-effects. You will then be more fully informed and able to decide which form of treatment is best for you. It should be your decision, not the doctor's.

Long ago, when a patient developed heart disease, it would take many years before he became disabled or died. Today, doctors have progressed. They can now accomplish the same result in a much shorter period of time, if we let them. They don't intend to; they mean well. But sometimes they don't know that they don't know. My fear is that 5,000 years from now, when anthropologists unearth all our bodies, they will discover everyone with a scar down the center of the chest. Inevitably they will conclude we were practicing some strange religious rite. That may not be far from the truth. It would not be inappropriate to compare bypass surgery to the mating of two elephants. It occurs at a very high level; it is accompanied by a lot of noise and trumpeting; and one does not know the results for a couple of years.

REFERENCES

1.Favalaro, R.J. Saphenous vein graft in the surgical treatment of coronary artery disease. *J Thorac Cardiovasc Surg,* 1969; 58: 178.

2. European Coronary Surgery Study Group. Long term results of prospective randomized study of coronary artery bypass surgery in stable angina pectoris. *Lancet,* 1982; 2: 1173.

3. Murphy, M.L., Hultgren, H.N., Detre, K., et al. Treatment of chronic stable angina: a preliminary report of survival data of the randomized Veterans Administration Cooperative Study. *N Engl J Med,* 1977; 297: 621-627.

4.Peduzzi, P. et al. Ten year incidence of myocardial infarction and prognosis after infarction. Dept. of Veterans Affairs Cooperative Study of Coronary Artery By Pass Surgery. *Circulation,* 1991; 83: 747-755.

5.CASS Principal Investigators. Coronary Artery Surgical Study (CASS): a randomized trial of coronary artery bypass surgery. *Circulation,* 1983; 68: 939

6.Braunwald, E. Effects of coronary artery bypass grafting on survival. Implications of the Randomized Coronary Artery Surgery Study (CASS). *New Engl J Med,* 1983; 309: 1181-1184.

7. Furberg, C.D., Friedewald, W.T., Eberlein, K.A. Proceedings of the workshop on implication of recent beta-blocker trials for post-myocardial infarction patients. *Circulation.* 1983; 67: Supp I: I-111.

8. Lewis, H.D. Jr, Davis, J.W., Archibald, D.G. et al. Protective effects of aspirin against acute myocardial infarction and death in men with unstable angina: results of a Veterans Administration Cooperative Study. *N Engl J Med,* 1983; 09: 396-403.

9. Schick, E.C. Jr, Liang, C.S., Heupler, F.A. Jr, et al. Randomized withdrawal from nifedipine: placebo controlled study in patients with coronary artery spasm. *Am Heart J,* 1982; 104: 690-97.

10. Hypertension Detection and Follow-up Program Cooperative Group. Reduction in mortality of persons with high blood pressure, including mild hypertension. *JAMA,* 1979; 242: 2562-71.

11.Kilip, T., Ryan, T. J. Randomized trials in coronary bypass surgery. *Circulation,* 1985; 71: 418-421.

12.Podrid, P.J., Grayboys, T.B., Lown, B. Prognosis of medically treated coronary disease patients with profound ST-segment depression during exercise testing. *N Engl J Med,* 1981; 305: 1111-1116.

13.Block, T., English, M., Murray, J. Changes in exercise performance following unsuccessful bypass grafting. *Am J. Cardiol,* 1976; 37: 122.

14.Peduzzi, P., Hultgren, H.N. Effect of medical versus surgical treatment on symptoms of stable angina pectoris. *Circulation,* 1979; 60: 888-899.

15. Dimond, E.G., Kittle, C.F., Crockett, J.E. Evaluation of internal mammary ligation and sham procedure in angina pectoris. *Circulation*, 1958; 18: 712.

16. Cobb, L.A., Thomas, G.I., Dillard, D.H. et al. An evaluation of internal-mammary artery ligation by a double-blind technic. *N Engl J Med*, 1959; 260: 1115-1118.

17. Selman, M.W., Experiences with the Beck Operation for coronary artery disease. *Diseases of the Chest*, 1955; 28: 1-19.

18. Sewell, WH et al J. The Pedicle Operation for coronary insufficiency. Technique and preliminary results. *Thoracic and Cardiovas Surg*, 1965; 49: 317-329.

19. Mulcahy, R., Daly, L., Graham, I., et al. Unstable angina: Natural history and determinants of prognosis. *American J Cardiology*, 1981; 48: 525-528.

20. Threading, U. et al. Effect of long term placebo therapy on angina frequency and exercise tolerance in patients with stable angina pectoris. *Circulation*, 1984; 70 (Supp 2): II-44.

21. Boissel, J.P et al. Time course of long term placebo therapy effects in angina pectoris. *European Heart Journal*, 1986; 7: 1030-1036.

22. G. Folli et al. Placebo effect in the treatment of angina pectoris. *Acta Cardiol*, 1978; 33: 231-240.

23. Benson, H., McCallie, D.P. Angina pectoris and the placebo effect. *N Engl J Med*, 1979; 300: 1424-29

24. Hueb, W., Bellotti, G., Ramires, J.A.F. et al. Two to eight year survival rates in patients who refused coronary artery bypass grafting. *Amer. J Cardiol*, 1989; 63: 155-159.

25. *Los Angeles Times*. March 27, 1988.

26. *Wall Street Journal*. May 11, 1990.

27. Glower, D.D., Christopher, T.D., Milano, C.A. et al. Performance status and outcome after coronary artery bypass grafting in persons aged 80-93 years. *Am J Cardiol*, 1992; 70: 567-571.

28. Kuan, P., Bernstein, S.B, Ellestad, M.H. Coronary artery bypass surgery morbidity. *JACC*, 1984; 3: 1391-7.

29. Grayboys, T.B., Blegelson, B., Lampert, S., et al. Results of a second-opinion trial among patients recommended for coronary angioplasty. *JAMA*, 1991; 268: 2537-40.

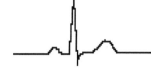

10.

THE ECONOMICS OF CORONARY BYPASS SURGERY

A $20 billion a year cottage industry.

F INANCIAL CONSIDERATIONS have a tremendous influence on whether a patient undergoes coronary artery bypass surgery. It is not whether the doctor needs to make a payment on his Mercedes next week. It is much more complicated than that. If the patient truly does not need surgery, or if surgery clearly will not benefit the patient, then I earnestly believe that most cardiologists will not recommend it. Having said that, I must emphasize again that economics has a great deal to do with the popularity of coronary artery bypass surgery, and more recently, coronary angioplasty, but in ways that may not occur to the reader.

In order to understand what happens, you need to consider the experience of the average doctor after he finishes his internship. He already has spent nine years after high school going through college, medical school and his internship and owes an average of $70,000. He is about 27-years old and still has four more years of residency training left. During this time, his salary will barely be enough for a decent living. This is especially true if the young doctor is married and has any children. It is not hard to understand why many of them select a specialty from which they know they will make a good living. Cardiology is such a specialty.

When one considers that medicine increasingly has become more of a business, it should not be surprising that fewer and fewer doctors are setting out on a career solely to help people. Undoubtedly this is an important factor in the loss of the personal touch and the old fashioned bedside manner. Cardiology is a lucrative profession, and is often considered as a business venture by a large proportion of young doctors.

We also need to consider the training young cardiologists receive at teaching institutions. Usually such training is taken at a university hospital. Traditionally such hospitals, like all hospitals, are in chronic need of operating funds. These institutions have long since learned that bypass surgery and, more recently, coronary artery angioplasty are a major source of funding. Indeed, most hospitals would probably go belly-up without the income provided from such interventions. Consequently, even though it is theoretically agreed that conservative medical treatment should be attempted first, surgical treatment is often urged upon the patient by the cardiologists and surgeons employed at the university hospital. It doesn't take long for the young cardiologist to develop a mind set on how to treat patients with chest pain.

The young doctor will have two options if he considers cardiology: one is to become a noninvasive cardiologist, the other is to become an invasive cardiologist. Noninvasive cardiologists must learn about many different kinds of tests and procedures. At the completion of his training, if he wishes to open an office, it will be necessary for him to purchase the noninvasive test equipment. This may cost several hundred thousand dollars. A technician will have to be hired to run the equipment, and it will have to be maintained, repaired and upgraded as new models become available. This can be a very expensive proposition and he can't expect to earn anywhere near the money that an invasive cardiologist makes.

On the other hand, if our young cardiologist decides to enter the field of invasive cardiology, he will spend most of his time learning how to perform angiograms and angioplasties. When he enters practice, he will not require expensive equipment because the angiograms can be done at most large hospitals. The hospital will purchase, service and maintain the necessary equipment and hire the personnel to operate it. In addition, the cardiologist will be handsomely reimbursed for the angiograms and angioplasties he performs.

It should be obvious why most cardiologists choose to confine their training to doing these procedures. And, since their training has been limited to these few areas, it is not hard to understand why they recommend angiograms as the first diagnostic test and angioplasty as the first treatment—it is the only way they know how to study a patient. Such technician-doctors conceal their narrow training by flaunting the incredible technology they command.

THE ECONOMICS FOR THE HOSPITAL

Prior to the introduction of high technology medicine, hospitals were dominated and run by doctors, almost all of whom were in private practice and had outside offices. There were exceptions, such as pathologists and radiologists who, because of the nature of their specialty, could work only inside a hospital. With the introduction of angiograms and bypass surgery, hospitals that wished to be on the cutting edge of technology were forced to purchase and operate very expensive, highly complex equipment for performing cardiac catheterizations and cardiac surgery. Such equipment required many skilled technicians and nurses and a sizable investment. Hospitals had little choice if they wished to attract to their medical staff the best doctors trained in the new diagnostic procedures and the finest surgeons qualified to perform expensive open heart surgery. Besides, other hospitals in their area already had the new diagnostic equipment. Unless comparable services were offered to their staff doctors, hospital beds would go empty, and they would lose patients and money.

It soon became apparent to the boards of trustees and the hospital administrators that optimum use of their expensive equipment could best be accomplished by hiring a full time cardiologist. After all, they were constantly seeing patients with chest pain in their emergency rooms. Traditionally, doctors in private practice had been called in to see such patients. Most were not trained in the new methods of coronary angiography and would not elect to use the hospital's equipment. On the other hand, if a staff cardiologist were called in to see the patient, his training and natural desire to perform angiograms would quickly put their new equipment to use, thereby helping to pay for its high cost. It was simply a way of amortizing their investment.

Soon advertisements appeared in medical journals offering attractive positions to qualified cardiologists interested in angiograms and starting up a cardiac surgery program. What an attractive opportunity for a newly trained specialist. After years of debt and subsisting on a minimal income, to be offered a ready-made practice, his own office and diagnostic equipment, and a very large salary was an irresistible offer. Hospitals were free to pick among the many candidates attracted by such opportunities. Of course, they were careful to select a cardiologist who was eager and aggressive.

Before long, business was booming. The hospital publicity department was quick to tell the local newspapers about their new capabilities. The hospital took pains to advise the doctors on its staff that these services were available, and that consultations could be arranged. Many of the local family practice doctors were only too glad to have their complicated heart patients taken off their hands. They were not trained to treat such patients who took a great deal of their time.

Within a few years, and with the increasing popularity of bypass surgery as the fashionable treatment for coronary artery disease, hospitals could hire more cardiologists and purchase more equipment. Soon bypass surgery grew to be their major source of income. High technology medicine was indeed very profitable. It also was moving forward with artificial heart valves, pacemakers, the surgical treatment of congenital heart defects, carotid artery surgery, heart transplant programs, coronary angioplasty, laser treatment of coronary artery disease, and the insertion of stents (tubes) within an obstructed artery. Each time technology moved forward, a cardiologist specially trained in the new technique had to be hired.

Obviously, the hospitals felt the availability of such highly sophisticated, costly equipment and specialists had to be brought to the attention of the public. They needed to attract more patients to pay for the equipment and continue the procedures that brought so much profit. Doctors needed to be informed in glowing terms of the benefits of the new techniques so they could send their patients to the hospital. Before long hospitals were holding cardiology symposia. Such meetings were usually held at plush resorts or hotels, and were widely advertised throughout the state, sometimes the nation.

Newspaper reporters were invited to these symposia and were granted special interviews with the cardiologists performing the new technology. The articles they wrote always interested a public that was anxious to learn about the latest treatments in medicine. Rarely did such articles detail the fact that such techniques were not the latest in medical treatment but the latest in medical experimentation.

Well-known speakers were invited to give lectures on the merits of a new type of diagnostic test, procedure or piece of equipment. Manufacturers of the equipment often supplied the funds for the cost of the symposia and transportation of the speakers. Of course, only those doctors favorable to the particular procedure or test were invited. These were the very same doctors who had published exaggerated claims in the past about their usefulness. It is of interest that doctors who had refuted such claims in published articles were never invited to these symposia.

In some instances, the procedure discussed in these meetings was a new and hazardous invasive technique undergoing investigation in only a few medical centers. In today's world, any information about a new medical treatment is rapidly made available to both the scientific community and public alike. The mere announcement of a new method prompted aggressive cardiologists, hospitals and medical centers to undertake the same technique. Their eagerness was not solely for the advancement of medical knowledge, but more for the future advancement of profits. Often the results were disastrous.

All this concentrated propaganda led the public to believe that the new method was already established and successful. No federal restrictions existed to limit the availability of surgical procedures, manipulative techniques and the like before they had been fully tested. Thus, the unsuspecting patient was often nothing more than a human guinea pig on whom aggressive and over-zealous doctors "practiced" medicine and buried their mistakes.

While all this was going on, hospitals were changing from non profit organizations to for-profit corporations. Not only did they seek to make a profit, but some tried to maximize profits. And yet, all they did was buy the equipment, hire a few select, highly specialized, narrowly trained, over-zealous doctors, and let nature take its course. Meanwhile, the cost of all this care was rising astronomically. In 1950, the total cost for health care in the United States was $13 billion, or 4.5% of the gross national product. In 1982, it was $322 billion, or 10.5% of a much larger GNP. In 1987 it reached $500 billion dollars, or 11.1% of the gross national product. In 1990, it was $666 billion or 12.2% of the GNP, and in 1992 it was $838 billion or 14% of the GNP according to the Health Care Financing Administration. In 1992 this amounted to $3,160 for every man, woman and child. Because so much of the cost of medical care tends to be concentrated in older individuals, without drastic changes, the Medicare system will be bankrupt within a relatively few years.

How many heart patients truly need all this heroic care? Nobody really knows, but according to a recent study conducted by the Rand Corporation in Santa Monica, there was "significant overuse" of every procedure studied. They estimated that $50 billion a year could be saved from the nation's medical bill. I think that figure should be many times higher.

Coronary artery bypass surgery has become, by far, the most common major surgical procedure performed in this country today, occurring about 390,000 times a year, or 1,500 surgeries per million people. In the United Kingdom with 57 million people, approximately 16,500 such procedures are performed each year, or 300 surgeries per million people.[19, Chap 7] We do nearly five times the number of bypasses they do. Yet, there is no evidence to suggest that patients in the United Kingdom receive poorer care than their American cousins. The death and heart attack rates in the two countries are similar. In other words, surgery neither prevents heart attacks nor premature death. The total cost of bypass surgery, with its accompanying screening tests and angiograms probably exceeds $20 billion dollars a year. The future cost of more frequent hospitalizations and more frequent heart attacks as a result of the accelerated progression of coronary artery disease caused by surgery probably adds a few more billion.

WHO PAYS?

If there is too much bypass surgery in this country, why isn't someone doing something about it? Well, who would that be? The cardiologist? Hardly likely; if he didn't do angiograms on all those patients he would lose a substantial portion of his income. The cardiac surgeon? Certainly not; he makes $250,000-$500,000 a year and would not like to lose all that money. The hospital? Goodness no; they would go bankrupt if they didn't have all those angiograms and cardiac surgeries to perform. The insurance company? After all they're the ones that have to pay for the cost of these things. No! Then doctors would complain that the insurance companies were restricting the practice of medicine. Besides, all the insurance companies have to do is increase their premiums. They can readily show the cost of medical care is much higher; everyone knows that. Of course, their profit is a percentage of their gross income; if their gross income increases because of higher premiums, so will their profits. Who then pays the cost? You, me, the patient, and the United States Government, who again turns around and taxes us more.

What if heart specialists were not reimbursed for angiograms? Would there be as many performed? Actually, that information may be surmised. In most large hospitals in metropolitan areas performing bypass surgery, about 1,500 angiograms are done each year. Assuming such a hospital services about 150,000 people, there is one angiogram performed for every 100 patients in the area. At a comparable HMO hospital servicing 300,000 people, and where the doctors are salaried, 200 angiograms are done each year, or one angiogram for every 1,500 patients. At the Royal Brompton National Heart Hospital in London, servicing about 2.5 million people under National Health Insurance, only 1,200 angiograms are done each year, or one angiogram for every 2,000 patients.

If it were merely an issue of unscrupulous doctors referring patients with recent onset of symptoms to cardiac surgeons, or if the surgery were not successful in relieving symptoms, the problem would eventually solve itself. However, many honest cardiologists, internists and general practitioners have been led to believe that bypass surgery is the best way to treat patients with coronary artery disease, and that medical therapy is not very effective. Surgery has become so fashionable that many doctors mistakenly feel it is the standard of care.

Doctors, as well as the public in general, have become victims of the knowledge and technology explosion. There are so many medical journals, reports, professional tapes, and meetings to read, hear, and attend, that physicians can literally spend all their time trying to keep up. Many scientific papers are worthless; they are written solely because doctors at major medical centers and medical schools must have articles printed if they wish to climb up the academic ladder. The more a doctor writes, the more prestige he commands. Because of the intense competition among journals, many papers are published when they should be rejected. With so many articles, there is insufficient time to read all of them carefully. Few physicians can afford the luxury of sitting down and reading a whole medical report from start to finish. They compromise by reading the summary. Poorly written material, those not supported by adequate facts, and those with unjustified conclusions, may be uncritically accepted as fact. The result has been the publication of massive amounts of misinformation. Claims as to the value, and safety of certain tests, procedures, and bypass surgery have been wildly exaggerated. Consequently, many cardiologists feel that bypass surgery is not only the preferred method of treatment, it is also safe. As we have seen from the discussion on the complications of such surgery, this is far from the truth.

While economics appears to be the driving force that fuels the increased use of high technology medical care, other non-economic forces also have a major impact. It has been shown over and over that hospitals with a high volume of coronary artery bypass surgery have the lowest mortalities. It takes years to develop the teamwork of highly skilled surgeons, surgical assistants, perfusionists, anesthesiologists, intensive care nurses, cardiologists, technicians, and other post-operative specialists. If you had to have bypass surgery, would you elect to have it done in a hospital that performed 40 cases a year or one that did 400 cases? In addition, Medicare and the insurance industry have decreed that in order for a hospital to be eligible for reimbursement for a given procedure, they must perform a certain number each year.

The same problem exists for the surgeon and the cardiologist. You wouldn't want to be operated upon by a surgeon who only did one or two bypasses a month. Nor would the hospital permit such a surgeon to operate in its operating rooms. Similarly, in order for a cardiologist to maintain his privileges to perform angiograms, a minimum number must be carried out each year. All this is understandable and even correct. But clearly, it forces everyone involved, doctors and the hospital, to encourage high technology care.

THE THREAT OF MALPRACTICE SUITS

The very forces that encourage high technology care and treatment also prove fertile soil for litigation. Imagine a scenario in which a 60-year old patient I will call Mrs. Black is referred to a cardiologist for evaluation of chest pain. Assume, too, that the doctor is reasonably conservative and feels that angiograms and bypass surgery are unnecessary. He makes this decision on the basis of the mildness of her pain, a normal cardiac examination, EKG and stress test. Our patient does not die, but she suffers a major heart attack shortly after her examination, and becomes seriously disabled. A friend of the family hears about Mrs. Black's misfortune. She, too, had similar symptoms but her doctor rushed her in for immediate angiograms and bypass surgery. Why hadn't Mrs. Black been treated similarly?

Our patient decides to consult an experienced malpractice attorney. He declares the cardiologist negligent for failing to perform all available diagnostic studies, and for failing to offer the patient the choice of bypass surgery. Wasn't it true, according to the newspapers, that this is the recommended treatment, and widely practiced throughout the country? Weren't over 1,000 such operations performed each day? Our patient sues.

Whether or not there was negligence (there was none), is less important than the knowledge that a suit was filed. This information quickly spreads throughout the medical community across the entire country. Regardless of the outcome of the suit, any doctor who sees a patient for chest pain is at risk of legal action if he fails to identify an impending heart attack. The fact that doctors are human beings and not prophets is irrelevant. The only defense against this situation is to perform a multitude of high technology tests, and to offer almost every patient surgery. Now, if the patient has a heart attack, or even dies, the doctor can say, "Well, we did everything we could." If there is legal action, at least the blame can be divided up among the cardiologist, the surgeon, and the hospital.

This kind of thinking encourages defensive medicine. Fear of litigation forces the doctor to order every available test and the latest treatment, even if its efficacy has not yet been fully established. The sad truth is that even though overdiagnosis and overtreatment is more likely to cause premature disability or death, the over zealous doctor is less apt to be sued than the conserservative physician who wishes to avoid costly and unnecessary tests and surgery. The impressive technology used on a patient discourages legal action in the vast majority of cases.

The factors I've discussed will have a profound impact on how a patient with chest pain is handled by the doctor. If he sees a general practitioner, an internist or noninvasive cardiologist who does not have a requirement to perform angiograms at regular intervals, that patient will be studied with noninvasive tests and will be treated with medical therapy.

On the other hand, if the same patient is seen by an invasive cardiologist, especially if that doctor is on the staff of a hospital or medical institution, he will almost certainly be submitted to an immediate angiogram. This will be followed by a recommendation for angioplasty or bypass surgery if he is in good enough shape for these procedures, and if he has insurance. Age is no exclusion. Some hospitals readily perform bypass surgery on patients in their nineties. When the choice is medical treatment or surgery, the latter is overwhelmingly preferred by the major hospitals, institutions and medical centers of this country.

In spite of the apparent popularity of aggressive forms of treatment for coronary artery disease, we have considerable evidence that coronary artery bypass surgery does not prevent heart attacks nor does it prolong life (except in certain rare instances). Furthermore, it is associated with a higher incidence of heart attacks in the post operative period, is followed by relief of symptoms in only 80% to 90% of patients, and is no more successful than medical treatment in promoting a return to work. Moreover, at least half of the patients who have bypass surgery have a return of their symptoms within five years. Indeed, we are beginning to see more and more patients who have had second and third repeat bypass procedures. The real villain here is not the doctor but the system that forces him to practice so aggressively. There are alternatives to surgery but unless the public demands them, the current high profit, high technology methods of treating heart disease will continue.

With the availability of so many drugs that can effectively re-lieve symptoms, as well as reduce the risk of a heart attack or premature death, it is inexcusable to pursue aggressive treatment before medical therapy has been tried. Too often the patient is the victim. He is made to undergo costly and unnecessary surgery, and even if he has no complications the surgery may still shorten his life without improving his heart condition.

Part III:

INFORMATION TO HELP YOU PROTECT YOUR HEART

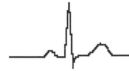

11.

ANGINA AND HEART ATTACKS

The circulation of the heart

W HAT DOES IT FEEL LIKE to have chest pain from coronary artery disease? A number of different conditions may cause chest pain; some are perfectly harmless while others are serious. Pain that is not originating from the heart is called noncardiac chest pain. The source of such pain may be from any structure within the chest cavity such as the esophagus (gullet) or lung. Pain also may originate from the nerve roots coming out of the spinal cord, or from the chest wall itself. Each of these sources of pain has its own characteristics, however, some general features of noncardiac chest pain should be brought to your attention.

The most common source of chest pains is the chest wall. Typically such pains are transient, last only for a few seconds, reach peak intensity immediately, are often produced by certain positions of the body, are relieved or intensified by movement of the chest such as breathing, are tender to the touch, and come and go for minutes to hours. Such pains tend to be localized to an area smaller than a golf ball. They are usually found in the region of the left breast rather than in the center of the chest where true cardiac pain is located. These kinds of pains can generally be ignored and will disappear within a few days.

Chest pain originating from within the chest may be from the lungs and is characteristically related to respiration. Breathing deeply intensifies the pain; not breathing causes it to disappear. Usually there are other clues that it is coming from the lungs; often the patient has a cough or an illness with a fever. The esophagus can produce pain not unlike that which comes from the heart; however, esophageal pain may last for hours at a time, is related to eating, and typically occurs while the subject is at rest rather than during exertion. In addition, the patient often has accompanying symptoms such as gas and regurgitation.

Pain that truly results from coronary artery disease is quite unique in both its character and behavior. We call such pain angina pectoris or angina for short. Many patients with angina are quick to emphasize that they are not having real pain. They describe it as a tightness, a fullness, a heaviness, a feeling as if their chest is in a vice, or a dull aching discomfort. As a rule, it is provoked by exertion, although it can occur at rest if the victim is experiencing a great deal of emotional distress. Usually it is confined to the center of the chest, and occupies an area about the size of a hand. Sometimes, it may spread across the whole chest. Occasionally it may radiate to the neck, jaw, left shoulder, and along the inside of the left arm. The feeling starts gradually; within 30-60 seconds it intensifies until the victim is forced to stop whatever he is doing. These symptoms often appear during exertion, after eating, in cold weather or under stress, and are particularly apt to occur when combined with movement of the arms. As a rule, the pain disappears within a few minutes of stopping the activity, although occasionally it may last longer. Slipping a nitroglycerine tablet beneath the tongue will relieve the pain in two to three minutes in most people.

The pain of a heart attack is similar in location, radiation and character, but is far more severe and prolonged. Such pain may be described by patients as crushing in intensity, or a feeling as "if someone were sitting on my chest." In addition to the pain, other symptoms are usually present in a heart attack such as nausea, sweating and profound fatigue. The victim commonly becomes very pale or ashen in color and may feel faint on standing up. You should suspect a heart attack with moderate to severe pain lasting beyond 15-20 minutes and in the absence of a specific cause. This requires immediate medical attention.

What you should do if you are having chest pain depends largely on whether you are having simple angina, or whether you are having severe pain because of a heart attack. Heart attacks are treated differently than angina, although the medications used might be similar. For the moment, let's put the subject of heart attacks aside and discuss angina more fully.

Doctors have divided angina into two categories. The first is stable angina, and the second is unstable angina. Stable angina refers to the predictable appearance of chest discomfort with a certain amount of exertion. For example, walking fast or up a slight incline usually produces symptoms, but they never occur when you are walking at a slow pace on level ground. It disappears promptly with rest, and its severity, duration, and precipitating causes do not change over a period of years.

In contrast, unstable angina describes two situations. In one, pain occurs in patients with no background of prior symptoms. In the other case of unstable angina, individuals with previously stable angina will experience changes in their symptoms, the pain may be more severe, last longer, or appear with less exertion than before. It also may show up under different circumstances. For example, sometimes the patient may feel the discomfort after eating, or while watching an exciting television program, or it may awaken him during the night, whereas in the past, it was only evident with physical exertion. Stable angina does not require urgent medical attention; however, unstable angina does, although it does not necessitate emergency care. Furthermore, the circumstances under which angina takes place also will govern how the problem should be treated. For example, chest discomfort that is noted only rarely, and then only with extremes of exertion, need not be handled with the same urgency as angina triggered by walking across a room.

Heart failure is sometimes confused with a heart attack by the public. The term heart failure is used when the heart has become so weakened by multiple heart attacks that the heart becomes greatly stretched, loses its elasticity, and is too weak to contract effectively. About 50% of all patients with heart failure die within just a few years of its appearance. In contrast, a heart attack is the lay term for a sudden obstruction of blood flow to the heart muscle, followed by injury or destruction of the muscle nourished by the obstructed artery. It is also called a coronary occlusion.

HOW CORONARY ARTERY DISEASE STARTS

What is this progressive obstruction of coronary arteries? How does it start, where is it located, and at what point does the degree of narrowing begin to interfere with blood flow? How coronary artery disease starts is not really known. What is known is that it begins at a very early age. During the Korean war, autopsy studies on young solders in their teens and twenties disclosed distinct evidence of coronary artery disease. In another study, supposedly healthy marines in their twenties and thirties, all of whom were runners, had angiograms as part of a research project. To the surprise of the investigators, a number of the soldiers had such severe coronary artery disease that they were ordered to stop running.

FACTORS WHICH ACCELERATE THE PROGRESSION OF CORONARY ARTERY DISEASE

Although, how coronary disease starts is a mystery, we are certain of many factors that accelerate its progression. Stress is one such factor. Cigarette smoking is another. Autopsy findings have disclosed that people who smoke have considerably more coronary artery disease than nonsmokers. In addition, when comparing victims of premature sudden death, nonsmokers die at an average age of 64 years while smokers die at an average age of 47. Hypertension is a third factor that will accelerate the development of coronary artery disease. People with high blood pressure always have more severe disease than those whose blood pressure is normal. This is one of the main reasons why patients with an elevated blood pressure are at high risk of a heart attack. In people with hypertension, the blood flows through the artery much more rapidly because the driving pressure is greater. This causes more trauma to the blood cells and aids in occluding the vessel.

In contrast to forces which accelerate the progression of coronary artery disease, certain factors can make you more vulnerable to the disease you have. Heredity, diet, weight and lack of physical exercise are just a few such factors. It is not uncommon to hear of several members of the same family who all have heart attacks at a relatively young age. In most such instances, the common denominator turns out to be hypertension. While you cannot choose your parents, hypertension can be treated to minimize the effect of your genetic influences. Similarly, excess weight puts an increase on the workload of the heart and intensifies the effect of any existing blood flow reduction. Recall how patients with angina can improve their symptoms with weight loss. Diet alone has not been proven to have any influence on the development of coronary artery disease, as we discussed in the chapter on cholesterol. The effects of exercise have been controversial. The prevailing view is that while a regular exercise program may not be beneficial to everyone, lack of exercise is harmful to all.

HOW VESSELS BECOME OBSTRUCTED

We now have a fairly good idea of the mechanisms leading to obstruction in the blood vessels. As blood flows through a vessel, some blood cells bump into the wall of the artery. One of the constituents of the blood is a group of cells known as platelets. When platelets are traumatized, they release a substance that causes the blood surrounding it to clot. We are fortunate that this happens, otherwise we would bleed to death if we cut ourselves. When trauma occurs to these platelets within an intact blood vessel, however, it eventually can create a problem. A minute amount of this clot-like material known as fibrin is deposited along the wall of a blood vessel, particularly where there are sharp turns and branches. At 100,000 times per day, 30 million times a year, the small quantity of fibrin eventually turns into a pile, and then a mound, and finally, the amount that is deposited is so large it can interfere with the flow of blood. The faster the blood flows, as with high blood pressure, the more quickly this takes place. Other material, such as cholesterol, is deposited there as well. Cells from the lining of the blood vessels migrate into this mound of material. Eventually the mound of fibrin, cells, and cholesterol becomes an arteriosclerotic plaque. It is important to note that only a small portion of the plaque has cholesterol in it, and, contrary to popular belief, cholesterol deposits alone do not plug off arteries.

In time, this plaque hardens and calcifies. If the residual opening in the artery is adequate for blood flow, nothing further is likely to happen, and the artery may never become obstructed. Sometimes, however, the plaque will rupture. When this occurs, a clot forms over the rupture site. If the clot fills the artery, it may cause sudden and complete closure of the artery. Usually, this will cause injury or permanent damage to the heart muscle nourished by the artery. We call this area of damage a myocardial infarction. The lay term is heart attack. If the amount of muscle damaged is large enough, it may cause the victim to die suddenly.

Interestingly, arteries that are 80% to 90% narrowed are less likely to close off than arteries that are less than 50% narrowed. The younger plaque is softer and more likely to rupture than a hard, calcified, older one. This is important because cardiologists are always rushing patients into surgery when they spy an artery that is 80% to 90% obstructed in the mistaken belief that a heart attack is imminent. At the same time they frequently ignore the artery that is only mildly or moderately narrowed. Could it be they are treating the wrong patients? A word of caution here. Vessels with a 99% obstruction will probably close off in the near future merely because blood can pass through such a narrow opening only at a very slow rate, and when blood flow slows down, it may clot. Thus, there is a more rational reason to operate on a patient with a 99% closure of an artery than one with 80% to 90% narrowing.

It is important to understand that as long as you are not physically active, blood flow will not be reduced in a coronary artery until it is narrowed by 75% or more. The more the artery becomes narrowed, the greater the pressure builds up before the restriction. This increase in pressure within the artery will maintain an adequate blood flow until the artery becomes so narrowed that the constraint of the opening exceeds the rise in pressure.

The narrowing of an artery may be compared to a four lane freeway in which one or two lanes are closed off. When traffic is light, the cars still flow. During rush hour, however, traffic must slow down because the freeway is now too narrow to accommodate all the vehicles. Similarly, with a narrowed coronary artery, when the heart is beating slowly at rest, the artery can accommodate the flow of blood needed. When the heart speeds up because its host is exercising or working, the heart muscle needs more oxygen to do the work. While the artery must be obstructed greater than 75% before blood flow is reduced at rest, during exercise only a 50% reduction may be necessary to interfere with the flow of blood. This is the principle on which the exercise stress test is based. Consequently, a patient with coronary artery disease may have a normal resting electrocardiogram, but it may become abnormal during a stress test.

WHY DO HEART ATTACKS OCCUR?

Almost one million Americans have heart attacks each year, and another half million die of various cardiovascular diseases. Yet, the public and physicians alike are remarkably ignorant as to why these events occur. No doubt a doctor who reads this will object to the term "ignorance," but might concede there is controversy over the causes of a heart attack. We do not understand why seemingly healthy people have heart attacks with no warning, while others, with known coronary artery disease, may go for decades and never have such an event.

We have known about chest pain due to heart disease for nearly two hundred years. We have known that the symptoms are probably due to narrowing of a coronary artery since the early part of this century. Yet, up until only ten years ago, it was believed that a coronary artery did not become obstructed until *after* an individual had a heart attack. Or does it? In autopsy studies on heart disease patients who die within 30-60 seconds from the onset of their symptoms, obstruction of a major coronary artery is found in only about 40% of victims. When the pathologist is asked why the patient died, often the attending physician does not get a definitive answer. We might be told there was severe coronary artery disease, or even that the patient had one or more heart attacks in the past, but a new heart attack, or obstructed artery cannot be found in most cases. Conversely, in autopsy studies on people who have died from noncardiac causes, a completely obstructed artery may be found, yet there is no record of a heart attack in that patient.

VARIABILITY OF CORONARY ARTERY DISEASE AND ITS SYMPTOMS

So far, one of the few things we know with certainty is the fact that coronary artery disease is highly individualistic and varies from patient to patient. One person with frequent and severe angina and an abnormal stress test might have normal appearing coronary arteries on an angiogram. At the other extreme is the marathon runner with severe coronary artery disease, but no chest pain at all. Also, the amount of physical activity tolerated by a patient with coronary artery disease may vary considerably. In spite of the fact that he has a fixed degree of narrowing of his coronary arteries, the patient's symptoms may show no constant limitation. In reality, on any given day, such an individual may be able to walk miles without any chest pain. Yet the next day, walking only a few blocks may provoke discomfort. Such capricious symptoms are extremely frustrating to both patient and doctor. Simply put, the patient doesn't know whether to feel good or bad. When he is able to walk several miles at a brisk pace without symptoms, euphoria is the likely response. On the other hand, when his chest pain occurs after a block, he feels he may not live much longer.

THE CORONARY CIRCULATION

Most physicians, when called upon to visualize the coronary circulation, bring to mind one of two views. The first, shown in

Figure 1, represents the heart's circulation as seen in the anatomy laboratory.[1] Two major coronary arteries arise from the aorta, the main artery exiting from the heart. The right coronary artery supplies blood mainly to the right side of the heart and the portion that comes in contact with the diaphragm. The left coronary divides a short distance after its origin into two branches. One branch supplies the front of the heart while the other nourishes the side and rear of the heart. The portion of the artery before the division is known as the left main coronary artery. Only rarely does this portion of the artery ever become obstructed, but when it does, it is a very serious matter. Most cardiologists feel a major obstruction of the left main coronary artery should be treated surgically. Since such an obstruction means almost certain death, that is not an unreasonable view.

In many respects, the branching of the coronary arteries is like the branching of a tree. Each branch becomes an entity unto itself. In the case of a tree, each branch is separated by a varying amount of space with no connections between branches. Such also appears to be the case with the coronary arteries. This impression of separate branches for each coronary artery is reinforced when one looks at a coronary angiogram. You will recall that the angiogram is created by injecting an x-ray opaque dye into a coronary artery and then taking high speed pictures as the dye passes down the artery. A typical angiogram is shown in Figure 2. Again, one sees arteries dividing and subdividing into smaller and smaller vessels with no connection between branches. You can see how if a coronary artery were completely blocked off, there would be a natural tendency to assume that blood could not get beyond that point.

ANATOMICAL OBSTRUCTION MAY NOT MEAN FUNCTIONAL OBSTRUCTION

The problem with this assumption is that it doesn't fit the facts. Commonly, an artery may be completely obstructed on an angiogram, yet there is no history of that patient ever having a heart attack. In addition, an echocardiogram reveals that the heart muscle fed by that artery, is functioning in a perfectly normal manner. How is this possible? There can be only one explanation, and that is the heart muscle must be receiving blood from a source not visible on the angiogram.

THE HEART'S MICROCIRCULATION

This brings up the question of how small a vessel can be seen by the angiographic technique? The angiogram can picture vessels down to one half a millimeter in diameter, or the thickness of the lead in a mechanical pencil. Any blood vessel smaller than this will be invisible. Ninety per cent of all the blood vessels of the heart are smaller than one-half millimeter. We call these tiny vessels the heart's microcirculation. Thus, the angiogram will not show any of the heart's microcirculation. Indeed, the angiogram can be likened to looking at a city from a high altitude. Usually, all one can see are the freeways. We know there are streets but they are totally invisible.

Now look at what the heart's circulation really looks like. Figure 3 represents the autopsied heart of a 17-year old male that was prepared by injecting the left coronary arterial system with a red-colored substance called vinylite, the right coronary arterial system with blue vinylite, and the veins with white vinylite.[2] One is struck by the network of small blood vessels that are not seen in Figures 1 and 2. Furthermore, if you look carefully, you will see many connections between the left and right arterial systems. This indicates a linkage between the two major arteries and a whole system of interconnecting vessels. If an artery is completely obstructed, blood can still find a path to the tissues it must reach, even though it has to go a different way. Such an obstruction may have only a minor effect on total blood flow. It can be likened to an accident that closes down a freeway; traffic will still get to its destination by taking a different road.

COLLATERAL VESSELS—THE HEART'S
ADAPTIVE RESPONSE

Keep in mind that Figure 3 is a normal heart not a diseased one. However, this microcirculation exists in everyone to varying degrees. It is well known that the body is endowed with tremendous healing powers and we are all capable of building new blood vessels when we need to. What happens when a coronary artery becomes occluded is quite unique. Upstream from the narrowed or obstructed arteries, new blood vessels sprout out from the wall of the artery much like buds from a branch of a tree. This takes place under a process known as angiogenesis (angio meaning "new vessels" and genesis meaning "birth of"). These new vessels grow and reinsert into the obstructed mother artery downstream from the obstruction. Alternatively, the new vessels can also connect up with a nearby healthy vessel. In either case, the heart creates its own bypasses. We call these new vessels the collateral circulation of the heart. It takes time for this to happen, and it isn't an instant process compared to bypass surgery. The advantage, however, is that the heart's own bypasses are not accompanied by the threat of dangerous surgical complications, they will last for life, and they are certainly less expensive.

Not only can we grow new collaterals between each of the coronary arteries, and from one part of an artery to another part of the same vessel, but new vessels can grow from blood vessels completely outside of the heart. Under certain circumstances, the arteries that supply the lungs will connect to the coronary circulation. I recall a postman who delivered mail every day by foot. He was studied because he had chest pain. His angiogram showed complete occlusion of all major coronary arteries. He refused surgery and continued at his job for many years. His body must have been actively growing new collateral arteries all the time.

It is worth emphasizing that the effectiveness of new vessel development is influenced by the amount of time available for growth. If the rate of narrowing of the coronary arteries is extremely slow, the increase in new vessels can compensate for the reduction in blood flow. In such cases, the subject may have extensive disease, and even an occluded artery, but never suffer symptoms or a heart attack. Conversely, if a coronary artery becomes acutely narrowed as a result of the rupture of an arteriosclerotic plaque, there is no time for the growth of new vessels. That individual may suffer a heart attack or sudden death.

It is clear that the network of blood vessels called the microcirculation provides alternative ways for the blood to get to its destination. This explains why so many patients with apparently severe coronary artery disease do not have symptoms, nor are they at high risk of a heart attack or dying in the near future.

Narrowed arteries show another wonderful adaptive mechanism when they enlarge in the region of the obstruction. Thus, if an artery is 85% obstructed by a plaque, and the plaque does not change in size while the artery grows larger to accommodate the obstruction, the plaque may now only take up only 60% of the vessel. This degree of narrowing is less than critical, and does not restrict blood flow at resting heart rates.

HOW BLOOD FLOWS WITHIN THE CORONARY ARTERIES

Figure 4 displays a cross section through the heart with its muscular wall and inner cavities. [1] Surrounding the heart is a tough, membrane-like sheath known as the pericardium. The reader should try to imagine the network of blood vessels seen in Figure 3 as lying within the muscular wall of the heart. These vessels have no protective muscular coat surrounding them whereas the larger arteries do. This allows the larger arteries to expand during the contraction phase of the heart's cycle and store the blood exiting from the heart. This expansion is distinct enough so that we can count the heart rate by feeling a pulse in the wrist. While the heart is relaxing and filling with blood for the next heart beat, the stored blood within the large arteries is pushed downstream as the artery contracts to its normal diameter. This insures a continuous flow of blood to smaller vessels throughout the entire cardiac cycle, rather than just when the heart is contracting. Accordingly, the smaller vessels do not have to store blood as the larger arteries do, since blood flows continuously. Unfortunately, the smaller the vessel becomes, the less it is protected by a muscular coat. In the smallest of vessels known as capillaries, the vessel is completely unprotected. Consequently, it is extremely vulnerable to even small changes in pressure *within* the wall of the heart. The value of a muscular wall surrounding an artery can be demonstrated quite easily by attempting to compress the radial artery in your wrist. The pulse (blood flow) can be made to disappear, but to accomplish this, considerable force must be exerted by pressing on the artery. In contrast, veins have no muscular walls. Therefore, it takes very little pressure to obliterate the vein and the flow of blood within.

HOW HIGH BLOOD PRESSURE INFLUENCES THE BLOOD FLOW IN THE CORONARY ARTERIES

When a patient suffers from hypertension, there is an increase in pressure throughout the entire circulatory system. This increase is also present within the heart's chambers. As I have previously described, the increased pressure is transmitted equally in all directions. Were it not for the thick, muscular heart walls and the pericardium which encloses the chambers, the heart would become acutely enlarged. Instead the pressure is transferred to within the muscle where it compresses the tiny vessels making up the heart's microcirculation. The effect is not unlike that which occurs when a blood pressure cuff is placed around an arm and inflated. The pressure within the cuff can effectively shut off the entire circulation to the forearm.

Similarly, the thin-walled vessels making up the heart's microcirculation will become compressed by the transmitted pressure from the heart's chambers, making it more difficult for blood to flow freely. The degree of obstruction to blood flow may be just as great as if one of the coronary arteries were partially obstructed. If this reduction in blood flow is great enough and lasts long enough, the patient will experience chest pain, a heart attack or may die suddenly.

UNDERSTANDING YOUR HEART—FACTORS OTHER THAN CORONARY ARTERY OBSTRUCTION MAY CAUSE CHEST PAIN

How can all this knowledge help the reader protect his heart? First of all, it is important to understand that just because you have chest pain and your doctor has discovered that you have coronary artery disease, this does not automatically mean the coronary artery disease is responsible for your chest pain. It is equally plausible that the coronary artery disease is *coincidental* and there is some other reason for your chest pain. Remember, you may have had your coronary artery disease for 30 to 40 years, but your chest pain has been present for only a few days or weeks. Why didn't you have symptoms last year? Remember, too, that coronary artery obstruction may exist without chest pain, that pain may occur in the absence of significant obstruction, that there exists a poor correlation between symptoms and the amount of disease, and the amount of pain present is not related to prognosis. Unless you have been tracked over time with various tests, you probably have no way of knowing whether your disease has progressed recently or not. Neither does your doctor—if he thinks so he is guessing.

This whole discussion would be pointless if there weren't a reasonable number of other causes of chest pain. By far the most common is hypertension. Because it is so common (one out of four older Americans), and because doctors almost never measure blood pressure during stress, it is easily overlooked. We will never know how many people have needless bypass surgery or angioplasty when all they really needed was blood pressure medication. The numbers must be staggering.

Frequently symptoms mimicking those of heart disease—such as chest pain, fatigue and shortness of breath—are caused by a silent urinary tract infection. Such infections are particularly frequent in older women, in men with prostate enlargement, and in patients with diabetes. Older women often have urinary infections because many have poor abdominal muscles and bladder support as a result of childbearing. This makes it difficult to completely empty the bladder. If residual urine is present bacteria may grow and cause an infection. With diabetes, this is even more likely to occur. Men with prostate enlargement also have difficulty voiding all the urine. In all of these situations, a reduced flow of urine causes the body to retain fluid. A significant portion of this excess fluid may be found within the circulatory system. Increasing the fluid content of a closed system, like our circulatory system, is like adding air to your automobile tire—a rise in pressure must occur. This increase in pressure is transmitted back to the heart's chambers, and from there to within the muscular walls of the heart. The microcirculation becomes compressed, blood flow is reduced, and chest pain occurs.

In such a patient, the symptoms may be deceptive; he may complain of chest pain but have no urinary symptoms. This is not a small matter. In today's climate of immediate surgery or angioplasty at the first appearance of chest pain, we can only guess at how many of these procedures were done unnecessarily when all a patient needed was an antibiotic.

Still another condition that can misdirect a doctor is the development of anemia. Anemia is relatively common in older patients. Most causes of anemia are not pertinent to this book, however, one, in particular, is worth commenting upon. Blood loss from the intestinal tract occurs often enough from peptic ulcers, erosion of the esophagus, diverticula in the colon, and even cancer. These diseases are common causes of anemia and should always be looked for in someone with cardiac symptoms. Anemia reduces the number of red blood cells that carry oxygen throughout the body as well as to the heart muscle. This reduction in oxygen can produce symptoms similar to coronary artery disease. Thus, the patient may have chest pain, exertional fatigue, shortness of breath, and palpitations. Obviously in such an individual, treatment should be directed at the cause of the anemia rather than at the heart.

A thorough physical examination, blood count, chemistry panel, urinalysis and other laboratory studies are mandatory in the careful evaluation of any patient with chest pain. There is no excuse for a brief examination followed by a recommendation for immediate angiograms. These precautions will help avoid one of the common errors in the practice of cardiology by technician-doctors. That error is the assumption that because a high technology test like the angiogram shows the presence of disease, then that disease is the cause of the patient's symptoms.

How can knowledge of the heart's circulation help you? If you have an obstructed coronary artery, you don't really have to worry that it will soon become completely blocked, nor will your other arteries quickly follow suit. You will probably not run out of blood vessels and die. This is nonsense. The heart has tremendous recuperative powers, and if you give it half a chance, you have an excellent probability that it will recover with the formation of new blood vessels. Perhaps you wont be able to run the 100-yard dash or play football with the kids or grandkids, but you don't need to—you can watch, which is better than dying in bypass surgery. There will be a great deal that you can do, but you will have to pace yourself, know what can cause symptoms, and avoid them whenever you can.

A diagnosis of an obstructed vessel doesn't mean that you will have a heart attack or die soon. Yes, that can happen, but in most instances it does not. How do I know that? Well, if everyone who had coronary artery disease died shortly after the onset of symptoms, we doctors would be out of business. We know that half the population will eventually die of heart disease. Another 25% have the disease but die of something else. Most people live a normal life span even with their disease. Chances are most of them don't even know they have it. The important thing is to not be frightened, you can live comfortably with it as long as you don't get talked into something by an aggressive doctor. Give Nature a chance—it usually does a pretty good job.

REFERENCES

1.Netter, F.H. *The Ciba Collection of Medical Illustrations*, Vol. 5, Heart. Ciba Pharmaceutical Co, Summit, N. J., 1969.

2.James, T.N. *Anatomy of the Coronary Arteries.* Harper & Row, Hagerstown, MD, 1961.

12.

HOW TO PROTECT YOUR HEART FROM YOUR DOCTOR

*If you are having symptoms, be careful;
the doctor you select may be more dangerous
than your disease.*

T HE WORLD has probably changed more in the past 25 years than in the previous 250 in terms of technology and scientific achievement, yet social attitudes and relationships between people remain fundamentally the same. Family values, trust among friends, honesty and integrity are the cornerstones of our existence. In the tumultuous world around us in which incredible changes occur at a dizzying rate, we tend to cling to these virtues as a survival tactic. While we may trade our car or TV for a newer model every few years, we do not change our feelings about people even over a lifetime. One of those primary relationships is often with our doctor. So trusting are we in physicians that their opinions and decisions are almost never questioned.

Nor do we find it necessary to learn about the disease that is bothering us—that is the doctor's job. Yet, if we wanted to purchase a new car we would research various models and their prices and select what appealed to us the most, and decide which we could afford. We would not let a car salesman sell us a $50,000 Mercedes when all we can afford is a $12,000 Ford. The decision would be ours, not someone else's. Why is it when we walk into a doctor's office, we put all these privileges on hold and let the doctor tell us what we need and how much we will have to pay for it, whether we need it or not, or whether we can afford it or not? Because we still cling to the image of the old fashioned doctor who can be trusted. Sadly, in many cases that image is fantasy. We can no longer depend upon a once fundamental truism—that the doctor is acting in the best interests of his patient. Forces beyond his control—the federal government, the hospital, the insurance industry, the pharmaceutical industry, the HMO or managed care plan for whom he works, and other members of the medical-industrial complex—have changed the way he views and treats patients. The patient is no longer an individual, but becomes a diagnosis that has to be treated by the rules of the health care system he belongs to. When a medical decision is made, that decision may be more for the doctor's or HMO's or hospital's benefit than for the patient's benefit. This situation will continue as long as the public fails to become more informed and passively submits to every doctor's recommendations. In return, doctors and the health care industry will continue to profit, often at the expense of the patient's well being.

What, then, should you do if you are concerned about whether you have heart disease, and whom should you see? The answer depends on whether or not you are having symptoms, and what kind of health care system you use. Let's begin by assuming you do not have any significant cardiac symptoms but you do have a positive family history. Furthermore, a close friend near your age recently had a heart attack without warning, and you don't want the same to happen to you. Finally let us presume you already have a family physician. Since you have no symptoms you've decided to turn to him for an examination.

In the absence of symptoms your most likely scenario will be that of underdiagnosis and undertreatment with the doctor taking your resting blood pressure, listening to your heart with an ordinary stethoscope and taking an electrocardiogram. He might even run some blood tests. By now you know the likelihood of this primitive type of examination discovering heart disease is small—no more than a 10% to 20% chance. When the doctor reassures you there is nothing wrong with your heart, what should you do? Thank him for his opinion, but tell him you would be more convinced if you had such additional tests as a stress test or an echocardiogram. If he says these tests aren't necessary because your examination was normal, ask him why there are so many other tests available to detect heart disease if the ordinary examination is that accurate? If you have other risk factors such as a stressful job, high blood pressure, an elevated cholesterol, a history of smoking, diabetes, or family history of heart disease, tell him of your concerns. Ask him to order those tests for you or refer you to a cardiologist. If the physician is in private practice he will readily agree to your request.

On the other hand, if you belong to a managed care program or an HMO, the doctor may refuse because the plan will not cover such tests in the absence of symptoms. At this point you will have to tell the doctor that you do not consider a simple blood pressure check, listening briefly to your heart, and the taking of an EKG an adequate examination. Moreover, you are well aware that serious heart disease may exist without symptoms and with a normal electrocardiogram. Inform him further that if you have to go to an outside cardiologist and find something really is wrong, you will hold him and the plan personally responsible. *You must change your views of medicine and doctors if you are to avoid being a victim of the doctor's limitations and your health care plan's restrictions.* Remember, you are the consumer and you have certain rights, even when seeing a doctor. You do not have to accept what you are told. All that is required is some knowledge of the disease you think is present, and the tests available for its detection. Otherwise you are apt to be the victim of underdiagnosis and undertreatment, and you will never know until it is too late!

If you do have cardiac symptoms then your worry will be at the opposite end of the spectrum—that of overdiagnosis and overtreatment. Who should you consult if you have symptoms of heart disease? You would be wise to know before symptoms develop. Once recurring chest pain appears, there is a sense of panic, and the victim is far more likely to accept the word of whomever is wearing a white coat. This is one of the reasons why so many patients passively accept whatever recommendations they are offered, including angiograms and surgery. They have no other physician to consult for a second opinion. If you live in a metropolitan area and have a family physician, make an appointment with your doctor within a few days of first experiencing the chest pain, palpitations, shortness of breath or fatigue you suspect is heart disease. Let him decide whether he wishes to handle the problem, or refer you to a specialist. The specialist need not be a cardiologist; an internist is perfectly acceptable. Your family doctor should know which specialist in your community is most likely to treat your symptoms medically, and which specialist is apt to rush you in for angiograms followed by angioplasty or bypass surgery. Alternatively, if you already know a cardiologist who treats most of his patients medically, only rarely advising surgery, then go see him. If you live in a rural area, a family physician may be the only one available. In any case, your family physician is best qualified to determine how your problem should be handled initially. Tell him of your concerns and let him know you are wary of invasive treatments and surgery. In the individual patient we have no way of predicting the most effective therapy. It seems rational to me that the treatment recommended first should always be the safest and least harmful, in other words, treatment with medication.

What kind of specialist you are referred to is less important than how you are treated. The important thing is that he be experienced and willing to treat you over an extended period of time before referring you for an angiogram. As a rule, it is possible to determine a specialist's qualifications by the amount of training he has had. While diplomas and training certificates verify that a doctor has received the necessary technical training, they will not tell you how good the doctor is, nor the reliability of his judgment. He may be an excellent technician capable of doing many cardiac procedures, but lacking in the art of clinical decision making and treatment. Nor do certificates tell you whether the doctor has compassion for your problem. Compassion is very important in a physician—at times, even more important than ability.

The first and most important principle to remember is that when a doctor suggests, or urges, you to have a test—any test, especially an angiogram—you have the right to ask about the risks. Specifically, inquire whether there is any danger the test could cause complications such as heart attack, stroke or even death. As a rule, in experienced hands, the likelihood of a major complication from an angiogram is quite low. One out of a 1000 might die, three to four could have a heart attack, one or two might have a stroke, three to four could have cardiac arrest with quick recovery with electric shock, and a few might have damage to the artery from the catheter. The problem here is that these statistics are from the medical literature. The complication rate of your specific cardiologist might be worse—it also could be better. So the first order of business is to insist that the cardiologist give you his statistics. While you are at it, you also might ask him how many he has done. If he only has a few hundred under his belt, he is inexperienced. A thousand or more is much better.

A common mistake is to select a doctor because he is busy, or has many patients in the hospital. It is a paradox of our profession that many potentially dangerous and even incompetent doctors are extremely busy. Medicine is the only profession I know where incompetence may be rewarded—if a physician takes poor care of a patient, and his disease gets worse, that patient will have to be seen more often, and will probably have to be hospitalized more frequently. It is easy to blame such results on the severity of the patient's disease. It is just as likely that the patient is receiving inadequate medical care. Yet, the doctor makes extra money seeing more patients at more frequent intervals. Never select a doctor who always has a large number of patients in the hospital, or whose office is always filled with people.

A comment is necessary here about hospitals and medical centers that always seem to receive a lot of publicity. Invariably, such institutions are the very ones guilty of acquiring the latest in diagnostic medical equipment and instituting the latest in medical or surgical treatment—prematurely! Since an unsuspecting patient may be harmed more with overtreatment by an aggressive doctor in a highly publicized medical center, it actually may be safer to stay away from such well known places. The more publicity a local hospital, medical center or clinic generates, the more suspect it should be. Doctors commonly refer their patients for diagnostic studies to such institutions. The mistaken belief is that because a particular medical center is well known, its patients will get good medical care. Unfortunately, that is not always true. Such centers may do good research, if you wish to be a human guinea pig, but the quality of their care may not be good at all, and may, in fact, be harmful.

View with suspicion any cardiologist who is employed full time by a hospital or institution to which you are referred. Hospitals depend upon the angiograms and cardiac surgeries generated by these doctors. They would not remain in the hospital's full time employment very long if most of their referrals were sent back to the originating doctor without an angiogram or cardiac surgery.

Be wary of any doctor, wherever he may be located, if he recommends a coronary angiogram anytime within your first few visits. A cardiologist often will tell a patient an angiogram is needed to determine how much disease is present. With this information he hopes to make a prognosis, as well as a decision on how you should be treated. This is deception, pure and simple, although not always knowingly on the part of the doctor. An angiogram is merely another test, not a crystal ball through which one can peer into the future. Doctors are human beings, not prophets, although some doctors tend to forget this. No test has ever been devised that will tell a doctor when a patient is going to have a heart attack, how long he will live, or how he should be treated. Accordingly, if the cardiologist insists upon angiograms, and you have not yet had the benefit of the more sophisticated noninvasive tests, politely decline. Tell the cardiologist there are noninvasive tests that will provide him with all the information he needs to know at this time. Make it clear to the cardiologist you are well aware the angiogram is not anywhere near the accurate test it was once thought to be, it will not predict whether you are going to have a heart attack, your prognosis depends upon the function of your heart, and not what the coronary arteries look like, and the coronary angiogram is not the best test to determine this information. Insist you will not even consider having an angiogram unless your chest pains are intolerable, and you are refractory to medical treatment. Let him know you are fully aware that these are the accepted guidelines for recommending surgery, and that the decision as to whether you have bypass surgery will be based upon your needs not his needs. Tell him, also, that occasional chest pain precipitated by exertion is not the equivalent of intolerable pain. Nor are a few brief visits to a cardiologist and the taking of a couple of cardiac drugs to be equated with maximal medical treatment, which often takes months. Inform him further it is your understanding that neither bypass surgery nor angioplasty has been found to be more effective than medical therapy. Furthermore, the side effects and mortality from these procedures are much greater than with medical treatment. If he feels differently, then his views are not supported by the available evidence.

If the cardiologist tries to make you believe you may have a massive heart attack and die while on medical treatment, tell him there's a much greater chance of that happening if you submit to angioplasty or surgery. Explain you would rather use your money for routine, noninvasive studies to track the progress of your disease. This will give him regular information concerning what is actually happening to your heart, and this knowledge can help determine his therapy. Advise the doctor you would prefer to have your treatment guided by serial, noninvasive testing over months or years than by a single test, such as an angiogram, administered at just one moment in time.

If you are hospitalized for a heart attack, and your cardiologist suggests angiograms, refuse to have the procedure. He may say it is the only way he can find out if you have coronary artery disease, and whether it is the cause of your pain, and that you might be a candidate for emergency surgery or angioplasty. Tell him there are other ways for him to discover if you have coronary artery disease, an angiogram will not determine the cause of your chest pain, and neither bypass surgery nor angioplasty is the latest in medical treatment for a heart attack but they are the latest in medical research. And tell that doctor, while you're at it, it is more dangerous to have emergency surgery for a heart attack, than the heart attack itself. Then ask your family to find you another doctor, preferably one that isn't so helpless without an angiogram. There is far less danger with this latter approach than submitting to bypass surgery within a few days of your first chest pains or a heart attack.

WHEN IS SURGERY APPROPRIATE DURING A HEART ATTACK?

Not everyone with a heart attack can be treated medically. Rarely, a patient may continue to have severe chest pain for many hours that cannot be relieved with multiple drugs in maximal doses. Even treatment with intravenous nitroglycerine fails to relieve the pain. Under these circumstances, angiograms and bypass surgery may be appropriate. Surgery during an acute heart attack may be desirable on a few other occasions. One such instance is when the victim is in a state of shock with an extremely low blood pressure. Blood flow to the brain can be so reduced that consciousness is impaired. In this kind of situation, a massive amount of the heart muscle may have lost its blood supply. This is called cardiogenic shock, and the mortality with medical treatment is exceedingly high. Recent evidence suggests that emergency angioplasty may salvage a significant number of these people by restoring the blood supply before irreversible damage occurs.

Another complication from a heart attack that requires emergency surgery is rupture of the heart muscle—usually the ventricular septum separating the left and right heart chambers. Prompt surgical repair usually will correct the problem. Occasionally the heart wall will rupture and this is almost always followed by immediate death. Rarely, the bleeding is contained by the membrane-like tissue called the pericardium. In this case, too, surgical repair of the heart's wall is life saving.

Still another major complication requiring urgent surgery is rupture of the muscle support to the mitral valve, the valve between the left atrium and the left ventricle. Rupture of this support muscle, which is called the papillary muscle, will be followed by massive leakage of the mitral valve and heart failure. Unless the valve is repaired immediately, the patient is likely to die within a very short time.

There are other instances when a patient is having recurring chest pain and medical treatment is not recommended. The most common example is the individual who has an obstructed aortic valve. This is the exit valve for the left side of the heart. Blood must go through this valve to enter the aorta—the main artery leaving the heart. Many older people develop calcification of this valve. As a result, it becomes stiffer and its motion is restricted. Ultimately, the restriction may be so great that the aortic valve is barely able to open. Since the coronary arteries arise from the aorta immediately above the aortic valve, coronary blood flow is restricted and chest pain may occur. Medication will not fix this— surgery is necessary and the sooner the better, because heart failure or sudden death is likely to occur in the near future.

HOW DO YOU FIND A NONINVASIVE CARDIOLOGIST?

How do you find a doctor who specializes only in noninvasive cardiology? This may be difficult since most cardiologists tend to prefer invasive procedures. Ideally, it is best to do this long before you have symptoms because it might take some time. The yellow pages of your local phone book might give you the information, particularly if your phone book lists doctors by specialty. If not, call the medical society of your county. If this fails, call the hospitals in your area, but first make sure each has a good reputation. Most hospitals have departments of noninvasive cardiology. Ask the hospital operator if you can talk with one of the technicians in the noninvasive laboratory. Once in contact with the noninvasive technician, ask for the name of the cardiologist who is in charge of the department. If all of the above fails, then ask as many of your friends as you can. Perhaps you can, at least, find the name of a good cardiologist. Even if he prefers to do angiograms, he is perfectly capable of ordering one or more of the noninvasive tests discussed in this book. Most cardiologists will respect your refusal of invasive studies, and will attempt to evaluate and treat your problem with other procedures such as an echocardiogram, a stress echo, or thallium perfusion imaging.

Many factors should go into the selection of a doctor, and into your decision to follow the treatment he recommends. It should be done with the greatest care because your life will be in his hands. Unfortunately, you may not always have a choice, either because your symptoms have developed too rapidly, or because you belong to a managed health care plan where physician selection is not an option. You should be aware any recommendation coming from a physician for a specific treatment is nothing more than his opinion. It is not a law that must be followed. If you do not like or agree with that opinion, then you don't have to accept it. A different physician may offer a different form of therapy. Keep in mind that the convictions of any doctor are based on the shared beliefs of other doctors. Those beliefs can change next month, or next year as new knowledge becomes available.

In times past, a patient could leave all medical decisions up to the doctor. Knowledge was limited, as were the options for treatment. Importantly, the rate of progress was slow enough so that treatment options were not apt to change from one year to the next, or even from one decade to the next. Nor were there external forces influencing the physician's decision. Today, these conditions no longer exist. The only solution is for every individual to have awareness of what is happening, and to take some responsibility for his own health. This means being informed about the various options for both diagnosis and treatment. Sometimes this is not possible. Not infrequently, the information is too technical. At the very least, if a treatment is advised by a physician, insist on being told about alternative forms of treatment with their risks and benefits. The doctor is morally, legally, and ethically bound to provide you with such information. You also have the right to ask for a second opinion, preferably from someone selected by yourself and not by the doctor you are seeing or the health care plan you belong to. Only after you have all these facts can you make an intelligent decision.

13.

HOW HEART DISEASE CAN BE DIAGNOSED AND TREATED EARLY

How a lethal disease can be tamed to become a benign illness.

ONE OF THE GREAT failures of the medical profession is its inability to find silent heart disease in apparently healthy people during a routine examination. We have no easy methods for detecting silent ischemia (reduced blood flow to the heart) before it is too late. Too, we need better methods to track the progression of heart disease in patients we have already diagnosed but who are not having symptoms that can be used as a guide. Current methods used in routine examinations to check the health of the heart, that is, the stethoscope and the electrocardiogram, are hopelessly antiquated. They are far too insensitive to detect early signs of heart damage, or to measure its progression. How then can we determine whether a patient is getting worse, better, or is unchanged on each follow-up examination?

NEWER METHODS USED TO DETECT
SILENT HEART DISEASE AND TO
FOLLOW ITS PROGRESSION

Over the past 20 years a number of noninvasive tests have evolved that do not require penetration of the skin, opening an artery, or the placement of a catheter within the heart. The doctors who do these procedures are known as noninvasive cardiologists. The beauty is, these tests are completely safe, most of them are relatively low in cost, and many can be performed in a doctor's office. Consequently, some of these tests can be used serially in the same patient to follow the progress of their disease. With information from these tests we can study the function of the heart and the blood flow to the heart muscle—the very things angiograms cannot do at all. The rest of this chapter will be devoted to a description of these procedures and the information they provide. A word of caution. While your first impulse is to think this will get too technical, and you don't really need these details, I urge you to read on. The information that follows will not be that technical, and someday you may need these tests to save your life.

THE EKG STRESS TEST AND THE
24-HOUR HOLTER MONITOR

Although the conventional electrocardiogram is not a very sensitive test for the detection of heart disease, it can be adapted to provide valuable information. Its primary limitation is that it will not show changes until *after* the heart muscle is injured. Consequently, the resting EKG rarely shows changes unless there has been a prior heart attack. In people who have regular episodes of chest pain or angina with exertion, but who have not yet had a heart attack, the resting EKG is likely to be normal, unless the tracing is taken while the subject is having pain. Since this rarely happens in a doctor's office, the electrocardiogram is likely to be normal.

The knowledge that specific changes may occur in the electrocardiogram while someone is experiencing pain led to the development of two related tests. One is the stress test, and the other is the 24-hour Holter monitor, named after the man who developed the monitoring technique. Both depend upon the principle that when there is an increased need for blood by the heart muscle for any reason—physical exertion, emotional stress, eating—distinctive changes will be temporarily displayed in an electrocardiogram if a coronary artery is narrowed. The recording has to be made during the activity to catch these fleeting changes.

The earliest attempts to accomplish this were made by an American physician by the name of Arthur Master. In the early thirties he recorded a patient's heart on an electrocardiogram immediately following a defined stress. That stress was walking up three steps and then down two steps a specified number of times during a three minute period. The older the patient, the fewer the trips. At the end of three minutes, the patient was connected to an EKG machine and a tracing obtained at one minute intervals. The Master's test, as it came to be called, was widely used by cardiologists of that period, and continued to be used for the next 20 to 30 years. A negative Master's test was equated with no heart disease, while a positive test meant coronary disease was present. The obvious limitations of the test were ignored. The first was that the EKG tracing was not obtained until after the patient had finished his exercise. As a result, changes that took place during exercise were missed. The second limitation was that many older or deconditioned patients were unable to walk up and down steps the required 30 to 40 times within a three minute period. Their fatigue ended the test before any EKG changes could occur. Consequently, the test was unable to detect a reduced blood flow to the heart muscle in many patients with coronary artery disease. Nevertheless, the Master's test was a valuable contribution to cardiology and ultimately paved the way for more modern stress tests.

In the fifties and sixties, the Master's test was modified in several ways. The first was to substitute a treadmill or a bicycle for the steps. Secondly, increasing amounts of exercise were carried out until the patient reached a predefined heart rate, depending upon his age. Lastly, EKG monitoring was maintained both during and after exercise. These modifications helped to uncover abnormalities that were only present while exercise was being performed. It did not solve the problem of fatigue and deconditioning.

The EKG stress test has remained the cornerstone of diagnostic testing for suspected coronary artery disease up until the present time. It continues to be used by most cardiologists as the only noninvasive test primarily because the technique is simple to perform, and the cost of the equipment is affordable. Unfortunately, time has established that for the average patient it is not very sensitive in the early detection of disease, and it is only moderately sensitive in patients with moderately advanced disease. In addition, many patients have alterations in their resting electrocardiograms, or are taking drugs that interfere with the interpretation of the changes that take place with exercise. While these factors seriously limit the stress test for diagnostic purposes, it remains a good test for predicting the patient's prognosis. Experience has shown that regardless of the severity of a patient's coronary artery disease, if his exercise capabilities are good, his prognosis also will be good.

The limitations of the treadmill stress test prompted other ways to uncover heart disease. One of those was the 24-hour Holter monitor. This required the wearing of several EKG electrodes on the chest for an entire day. Originally, the electrodes were connected to a tape recorder and the entire apparatus was strapped around the patient's body. At the completion of the test, the tape was played back on a special recorder so that the cardiologist could review every heart beat in the 24-hour period. This was not a small undertaking considering that there might be 100,000-120,000 heart beats per day. Today a microchip records all the patient's heart beats over a 24-hour period. The information for each heart beat is processed, interpreted, and later stored on a floppy disk. Upon completion, the floppy disk is placed in a microcomputer and a summary is printed out. Any portion of the original analog information can be displayed at will.

The Holter monitor has turned out to be a valuable noninvasive test particularly suitable in patients unable to perform a stress test. It also is useful in subjects who have rhythm disturbances of their heart beat that might only occur a few times a day. Its most valuable contribution has been in the detection and treatment of patients with transient episodes of reduced blood flow to the heart muscle, a phenomena known as silent ischemia. This will be discussed in more detail in the next chapter.

THE APEXCARDIOGRAM

One of the most valuable and least expensive of all the noninvasive tests that can be obtained in an office is the apexcardiogram. This procedure depends upon the principle that when a subject lies on his left side, the heart will fall to the left side and come in contact with the chest wall in the general vicinity of the nipple in the male. Try this experiment: find a subject, preferably a man, and have him lie on his left side. Place your right hand about two or three finger-widths below the nipple, in the direction of the bed. In most subjects with normal hearts, it is possible to feel an impulse against your hand about the size of a quarter or fifty-cent piece. If the heart is abnormal, or if high blood pressure is present, then the impulse area will be much larger. Now, take your other hand and place it upon the radial pulse in the subject's right wrist. With a little practice, you will soon discern that the radial pulse occurs almost simultaneously with the impulse against your right hand. Actually, the pulse occurs about 0.1 second after the cardiac impulse because it takes that long for the pulse wave to reach the artery in the wrist.

Unfortunately, with our hand we can feel the pattern over the heart only during its contraction. By placing a recording device known as a transducer over the cardiac impulse, the pattern of motion of the cardiac impulse can be translated into waves on an oscilloscope and recorded. That pattern is called an apexcardiogram. The name comes from the fact that cardiologists call this impulse the apex beat, presumably because it was originally thought to be originating from the apex of the heart.

Clinical experience with the apexcardiogram throughout the world for the last twenty-five years has established that it is extraordinarily valuable in reflecting three things—how well the heart contracts, how well it relaxes, and whether sections of heart muscle are in jeopardy because an artery is obstructed. It is remarkably sensitive in the early detection of heart disorders, and is one of the few tests in cardiology that gives reliable information about the filling of the heart. This is extremely important because when the heart has been damaged, or its blood supply impaired, it becomes stiffer. In much the same way that some balloons are harder to inflate than others, hearts that are diseased are harder to fill, and produce distinctive changes in the apexcardiogram. Since it is quite easy, inexpensive and safe to repeat the apexcardiogram at each patient visit, daily if the patient is in the hospital, it provides directional information about heart function over a period of time. In other words, it will tell us whether someone with heart disease is getting better, worse, or is unchanged. The apexcardiogram also may be used after stress, either with a hand grip stress test or following exercise. It often will show abnormalities, both in the contraction of the heart muscle, and in the filling of the heart, before other tests show any changes, and long before the appearance of symptoms. Unfortunately, most modern cardiologists no longer do apexcardiograms on patients—they can make more money doing angiograms.

LISTENING TO THE HEART WITH
MODERN INSTRUMENTS

The diseased heart often generates abnormal sounds that are inaudible with the stethoscope because of their very low frequency. High frequency heart murmurs also may be missed because they are too faint. Modern instruments for listening to the heart can amplify these low or high frequency sounds, much like the base and treble control of a stereo system. More precise control can be obtained with a graphic equalizer that selectively amplifies certain groups of frequencies. Subaudible low frequency sounds also can be visualized on the screen of an oscilloscope, enabling doctors to see what they cannot hear. This is important because, unlike the human ear, the recording microphone is able to detect low frequency sounds coming from the heart.

The presence of these abnormal sounds or murmurs usually means that the function of the heart is abnormal, or that heart disease is present. If, over a period of time, the sounds increase in size or loudness, the patient's disease is getting worse. Conversely, their disappearance after a patient takes heart medication, means the drug is allowing the heart to contract better.

RECORDING HEART SOUNDS—
THE PHONOCARDIOGRAM

An obvious limitation of the stethoscope, even the more sophisticated ones, is the fact that it leaves no record of what the doctor heard. As a consequence, he cannot possibly remember what a specific patient's heart sounded like months before. Thus, he has no objective way of comparing these heart sounds or murmurs. One of the least used noninvasive tests entails the recording of heart sounds on a phonocardiogram. A phonocardiogram gives the doctor a permanent record of the amplitude and frequency of the patient's heart sounds, as well as capturing any abnormal sounds that cannot be heard with a stethoscope. Evaluating the change in the phonocardiogram is an effective way of following the progress of the patient's disease and its response to treatment. It is also a potential way of detecting new disease in a patient without symptoms.

THE ECHOCARDIOGRAM

Another type of procedure that is highly successful in detecting early heart disease is the echocardiogram, or an ultrasound examination of the heart. It is really a form of sonar wherein a sound beam is focused inside the chest. The sound waves are translated into images that are then sent to a screen or stored on video tape. This test shows the doctor the chambers inside of the heart and the muscular walls that surround those chambers. As a result he can analyze the motion of the heart muscle as it contracts and relaxes. If a portion of the heart's muscular wall fails to move, it indicates this area of the heart has been damaged from a heart attack. If, however, it moves partially, then the blood flow to this area is reduced rather than completely cut off.

Not only is the echocardiogram useful for detecting heart disease, it is also helpful in guiding treatment. For example, if we see impaired motion of one of the muscular walls is hindering the heart's ability to contract, and that contraction improves following the administration of a drug such as nitroglycerine, we can conclude the drug helped and the patient would benefit from its regular use. Permanently damaged muscle will not show an improvement in motion after nitroglycerine. Consequently we have gained information from this test about the health of the heart muscle as well as a good idea as to what treatment will or will not work.

With an echocardiogram the doctor can accurately measure the thickness of the heart muscle and the dimension's of the heart's chambers. This is of considerable help in detecting high blood pressure, and following its progression. For example, if you have borderline high blood pressure of 140/90, there is no practical way of knowing whether this is an average blood pressure for you or not. An ambulatory blood pressure monitor could reveal your pressures over a period of time, but we wouldn't be sure whether the values are constant or merely reflect your activities and stress levels on that particular day. An echocardiogram can provide a clue to your long term blood pressure. The heart is a muscle and responds to an increased workload like any other muscle, by growing bigger. Consequently, the heart's chambers will be enlarged if your blood pressure is elevated for a significant length of time. An echocardiogram will demonstrate this, greatly simplifying the problem of diagnosing and treating an individual with borderline high blood pressure. If the blood pressure is not brought under adequate control, successive echocardiograms will show a progressive enlargement of the heart's chambers. In contrast, successful treatment will be followed by a decrease in chamber dimensions.

One of the major limitations of a typical examination, regardless of the test being used, is that it is performed with the subject at rest. Studying the function of the heart is not much different from checking the performance of an automobile or any other piece of equipment. If you are looking for a new car, a certain amount of information may be acquired merely by looking or listening to the motor idle. Few of us would buy a car without taking a road test. Intuitively, we all recognize that performance is the ultimate test.

For this reason, various types of stress tests using the echocardiogram have evolved in an attempt to discover heart disease when the resting test fails to disclose any abnormality. One such test is called the hand grip stress test and takes only one minute to perform. After a baseline recording is obtained, the patient squeezes a device known as a hand grip dynamometer. If one isn't available, a half inflated blood pressure cuff or a tennis ball will do. The trick is for the subject to squeeze as hard as possible for one minute. This simple effort is capable of creating an abrupt increase in workload for the heart, and along with it, an immediate requirement for more oxygenated blood. If obstructive coronary artery disease is present, and of sufficient degree, the blood supply to the muscle may be adequate at rest, but inadequate if the heart has to work harder. Accordingly, the muscle will be unable to perform the extra work, there will be discordance between the amount of motion of the two walls of the ventricle, and this can be readily visualized on the echocardiogram.

The heart can be stressed to only a limited degree with a hand grip test. Consequently, more vigorous forms of stress can be used to make the heart work harder. Commonly, the patient peddles a bicycle ergometer during an exercise stress echocardiogram. Many noninvasive laboratories have the patient lie down to pump the bicycle. This makes it easy to image the heart during exercise. If one of the two walls of the contracting heart is not receiving enough blood, the inequality of motion usually can be seen on the echocardiogram.

Some patients are unable to exercise, so doctors use certain drugs to speed up their heart rate. Currently there are three such drugs used by noninvasive cardiologists. They are Persantine,

Dobutamine and adenosine. The drugs are given in an intravenous drip with the dosage being gradually increased. Since the heart muscle requires more oxygen when the heart rate increases, and therefore, a higher rate of blood flow, any differences in the amount of movement of the muscular walls, or of the pattern of contraction, will indicate significant obstructive coronary artery disease.

In addition to its use in patients with coronary artery disease, the echocardiogram is invaluable when the patient has suffered damage to any of the heart's four valves. Whenever a heart valve is diseased sufficiently to interfere with the flow of blood entering or leaving the heart, a heart murmur is produced. Frequently it is difficult to locate which valve is producing such a murmur in much the same way the source of a car noise is often hard to identify. The transmission of the sound distorts its origin. Echocardiography will usually show which valve is damaged. In addition, with the introduction of the echocardiogram, the treatment of valvular heart disease totally changed. One of the major problems in the care of such a patient is in deciding when the damaged valve should be replaced with an artificial one. If the surgeon replaces the valve too soon, that patient is in danger of having to undergo two or even three such operations during his lifetime because artificial valves usually last only 10 to 15 years. However, if the surgeon waits until the patient develops symptoms, the heart will have become very enlarged. Such a heart cannot contract very well, and heart failure quickly follows. In such circumstances, even if the damaged valve is replaced, the heart has become stretched out, and has permanently lost its elasticity. Such patients do very poorly, and die within a few years. Prior to the use of the echocardiogram, the only guide that physicians had was an electrocardiogram and a chest x-ray to show the heart size. Neither test was particularly reliable; consequently, many patients had their valves repaired when it was too late. The operative mortality was very high (25%), and survival poor after surgery. Now with the use of echocardiograms, the dimensions of the heart can be tracked accurately. As soon as it becomes apparent that heart size is increasing beyond a certain limit, the valve can be replaced, even if the patient still hasn't developed any symptoms. The results have been striking—operative mortality has been reduced to 5%, and post-operative survival is excellent.

COLOR FLOW DOPPLER

Another kind of ultrasound examination is the color flow Doppler. This test depends upon the change in frequency that takes place when a sound wave leaves a moving object. For example, an approaching train sounds different from one which is moving away from you. In the former instance, the sound waves leaving the train are closer together because the train is going in the same direction as the sound waves. They have a higher frequency than when the train and the sound waves are traveling in opposite directions.

This principle can be used to determine the speed of a moving object, in this case the flow of blood as it enters and leaves the heart. By checking the frequency of the sound waves, it is possible to determine whether the blood is flowing forward or backward. This is of great practical importance in determining the source of a heart murmur. The Doppler machine has been engineered so that the sound waves reflected from blood entering the heart are visualized as red. Conversely, the sound waves reflected from blood leaving the heart are blue. When the color flow Doppler is applied to an echocardiogram, the doctor can see red blood entering the heart during its relaxation phase. This represents the newly oxygenated blood. When the heart contracts, blue blood can be seen exiting the heart and entering the aorta, if the heart is normal. However, if the mitral valve fails to close properly, leakage will occur when the heart contracts, and blue blood will enter the left atrium. It is not only the wrong color inside of this chamber, it is coming from the wrong direction. The examiner immediately knows there is leakage of the mitral valve. Many times the patient may have a murmur too faint to detect, however, the color Doppler will not be fooled by this silence. Such information is of major clinical importance in the diagnosis and treatment of a number of heart conditions.

SYSTOLIC AND DIASTOLIC TIME INTERVALS

Another type of test that can be performed in a doctor's office is a procedure that measures the systolic and diastolic time intervals. Systole refers to the contraction phase of the heart's cycle, while diastole refers to the relaxation phase of the cycle. It is possible to measure the duration of each phase of the heart's cycle within an accuracy of only a few milliseconds (one millisecond is 1/1000 of a second). For example, we can measure how long it takes for the heart to build up enough pressure so that blood can be ejected into the circulation. This might be likened to how long it takes for an automobile to go from zero to 60 miles-per-hour. That duration of time is a measure of the car's performance. The same is true for the heart. Normally it requires about 70-80 milliseconds for the pressure to rise sufficiently so that blood can be ejected rapidly into the circulation. If it takes 125 milliseconds, then clearly there is something wrong, and the most likely reason is the presence of coronary artery disease. Similarly, if 375 milliseconds are required for blood to leave the heart during its contraction phase when it only should take 325 milliseconds, then there is a reason for the delay. It may be that the heart muscle is diseased and is unable to contract as rapidly as it once did. Alternatively, the exit or aortic valves may be obstructed so it takes longer for the blood to get out. Or there may be a stress related increase in fluid in the circulatory system, and it requires more time to eject the increased volume of blood with each heart beat. In any case, something is wrong. Measurement of the systolic and diastolic time intervals can be done easily, and at a low cost. Accordingly, it is very useful for both the detection of heart disease and for following its progress.

RADIOACTIVE IMAGING TESTS

A variety of radioactive imaging procedures are available and are useful in detecting the presence of coronary artery disease, or the presence of a prior heart attack. The most commonly used test is the thallium perfusion study. Thallium is a substance with a special affinity for heart muscle cells. In radioactive imaging procedures, a radioactive solution is injected into the blood and, from there the radioactive particles distribute themselves throughout the heart muscle. A recording instrument that detects radioactive material will form an image of the distribution of that material. The picture that results is a reflection of the actual circulation within the heart's muscular walls. This kind of test tells us what the angiogram cannot because it is not limited by vessel size.

Generally, the distribution of all radioactive material within the heart is uniform. If, however, the blood supply is blocked in an area of the heart, or if the heart muscle cells have been damaged or destroyed, then little or no radioactivity will have been able to reach this area. It will show up as an empty spot if there is no functioning tissue, or it will be much lighter than other areas of the picture if there is only some functioning tissue.

This test can be conducted while the patient is exercising to identify problems that won't show up at rest. This type of test is called an exercise thallium perfusion study. As with all the other noninvasive tests, thallium perfusion studies not only can be used for diagnostic purposes, but to follow the course of a patient's disease and to make decisions about treatment.

Thallium perfusion studies have several limitations. The first is that it requires radioactive material and rather sophisticated equipment to do the test. Thus, the cost is high ($800-$1,000) and its complexity limits its use when the doctor needs a quick answer. Too, it is impractical to use frequently to follow the progress of a patient's disease. Nevertheless, it is an extremely valuable test, is widely available, and is far preferable, less expensive, and safer than a coronary angiogram.

A word of caution is necessary here. Some cardiologists will combine a thallium study with an angiogram to determine whether an obstructed coronary artery is restricting blood flow. The problem with this approach is why do the angiogram if decisions are to be made from the noninvasive test? A positive outcome often leads to an immediate recommendation for angioplasty or bypass surgery. Sometimes the doctor will even recommend surgery when the results of the test are negative on the grounds that blood flow will surely be reduced in the future. In the former instance you should remember that if you give Nature a chance, and with the help of medications to increase blood flow, often the circulation to the heart will be restored with the natural development of new vessels. In the latter instance, the doctor has assumed the role of a prophet and his advice should be so considered—no test will allow him to make such a prediction.

POSITRON EMISSION TOMOGRAPHY

One of the current problems in cardiology is distinguishing injured heart muscle from dead or scarred tissue after a heart attack. The damage may not be severe enough to destroy the muscle but may leave it receiving barely enough blood to remain alive. It is certainly unable to function normally. We call such heart muscle hibernating myocardium (myocardium means heart muscle). On an angiogram the artery going to the hibernating myocardium may appear completely obstructed. On imaging the area with an echocardiogram or a thallium perfusion study, the study may show no function; therefore, the area is usually presumed to be dead. In fact, it may not be.

The test used to make this distinction is called a PET study, which stands for positron emission tomography. This is another form of radioactive imaging; however, in this situation we do not want to depend on blood flow to the heart muscle to distribute a radioactive substance, because the flow may be too small. Instead, we look at the metabolism of certain substances within the heart cell such as glucose, nitrogen and ammonia. Radioactive substances are used that will be incorporated directly into the cells of the heart muscle. If the cell is alive, the metabolism of the substance will become evident, and the resulting radioactive emissions can be detected.

The practical application of a PET test lies in cardiac patients who are doing poorly either because of severe impairment of blood flow or because of prior multiple heart attacks. Such a patient will not do well, despite treatment with drugs. One of the guiding principles of medical treatment is that once a tissue or an organ is dead, it cannot be brought back to life. A patient who is thought to have segments of dead heart muscle is apt to be given inadequate treatment because the doctor believes nothing further can be done. In such cases, a PET study may show viable heart muscle. Bypass surgery in such a patient may provide enough new blood supply to allow the hibernating myocardium to function, if not normally, at least well enough to improve the quality of life.

MAGNETIC RESONANCE IMAGING & CINE MAGNETIC RESONANCE IMAGING

Over the past ten years magnetic resonance imaging (MRI) has become one of the most impressive imaging tests ever introduced into clinical medicine. Whereas an x-ray only provides a silhouette of a structure or organ, an MRI enables us to see inside that organ. For example, if an individual fractures his skull and has bleeding on the surface of his brain as a result (subdural hematoma), an x-ray will readily image the fracture but will not be able to picture the bleeding. If a hypertensive patient has a stroke it will not be detected by an x-ray. In contrast, an MRI will allow doctors to see both the subdural hematoma and the area of the brain where the stroke took place because of its ability to visualize the tissues inside an organ.

An MRI test will permit us to see the inside of the heart allowing us to visualize the character of the muscle, its chambers, their dimensions and geometry, the valves, and even the blood inside the arteries. An MRI test can determine whether a section of the heart muscle has been damaged by looking at the difference in thickness and color of the muscle. If a valve is damaged or has calcium deposits, it will be evident, and if a clot or a tumor is residing within the heart, it will be apparent.

A special adaptation of MRI imaging is a procedure called cine magnetic resonance imaging. Although the MRI technique is capable of taking only static images, by taking those images every 50 milliseconds throughout the cardiac cycle, it is possible to sequence these multiple images together in the same way as animating a cartoon. The cartoonist creates multiple pictures of a person or animal, each slightly different than the preceding one, and each representing the next step in an act of motion. When pictures are viewed rapidly in sequence, they appear to be moving. In the same way, the static images obtained with the MRI at successive intervals, will allow us to image the heart contracting and relaxing. A discordance in the contraction pattern between two walls indicates impairment of blood flow or damage to the muscle. The great advantage of cine magnetic resonance is its ability to image the heart in all views, even views that are difficult to see with other techniques. Also, the pictures look like a heart—it is what a doctor would see if the heart were cut open at an autopsy. It is not a sonar image on a screen or a bunch of squiggly lines that have to be interpreted. The disadvantages of this technique lie in its reliance on highly sophisticated technology and trained personnel, as well as the logistics of transporting a sick patient to a MRI facility, all of which lead to a high cost. Nevertheless, ultimately the logistics and technology will be simplified so that it can be used more routinely.

IMPACT OF THE NONINVASIVE TESTS

The impact of noninvasive tests on the diagnosis and treatment of heart disease has been enormous. In much the same way as a microscope allows doctors to see things that cannot be viewed with the unaided eye, so have these new tests opened up modern ways to diagnose and treat heart disease. Early detection of disease many years before symptoms or complications appear has permitted early treatment. Noninvasive tests have been responsible for a drastic decline in heart attacks and deaths from heart disease, as well as the need for such heroic approaches as bypass surgery or angioplasty. This is true preventive medicine.

Similarly, the repeat use of noninvasive tests as the patient is being followed, has permitted the early discovery of recurrent flare-ups of the patient's disease. In my experience, the routine use of noninvasive tests has uncovered changes in the function of the heart long before the occurrence of unstable angina. Failure to promptly adjust the patient's medical program in these situations, has been followed by progression of the patient's disease. In contrast, adding new medications, or increasing the dosage of existing drugs has avoided such progression in most cases. In many instances, it has been possible to uncover a coexisting condition such as a silent urinary tract infection, anemia or the effects of stress. The detection and treatment of these conditions has prevented the appearance of new symptoms, a heart attack, and even unexpected death. The result has been that a previously lethal disease has been tamed to become a relatively benign illness, and often the patient can live a normal life span.

Noninvasive tests of the heart can revolutionize the field of cardiology in both diagnosis and treatment. Before that can happen, the public must be made aware of their existence, and insist that one or more of these procedures be utilized on a regular basis in their care. Only then will the more dangerous procedures, such as angioplasty and bypass surgery, be relegated to the few cases that really justify them.

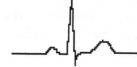

14.

DRUGS USED TO TREAT HEART DISEASE

Why they are necessary.

MANY DOCTORS have had the privilege of serving their country in the armed forces; I was one of them. Because of my special training in cardiovascular physiology, I had the further honor of being assigned to the Faculty of the United States Air Force School of Aerospace Medicine at Randolph Field in Texas not far from San Antonio. At that time the Air Force was concerned about problems facing flyers in the upper levels of our atmosphere such as hypoxia (lack of oxygen), hyperventilation (over breathing), the effect of G forces and other stresses. Two problems in particular caught my attention, both of which involved the same challenge.

The first and immediate problem was the number of unexplained aircraft accidents with high performance planes. When no mechanical cause could be found, it was assumed these accidents were the pilot's fault. Indeed, the Air Force command in Washington had a high suspicion that many of the pilots had had heart attacks under the intense stress of flying such vehicles. It is likely that this assumption came about because of evidence of coronary artery disease in the deceased pilots. Recall that arteriosclerosis also was found in young American soldiers who died in Korea. The presence of unsuspected coronary artery disease in pilot victims must have distressed the high brass because it had not been detected on their annual examinations. All pilots had been put through an intense physical examination and a stress test every year. Anyone found to have coronary artery disease was immediately grounded. Many a pilot's flying career came to a sudden halt because of some insignificant change in his annual electrocardiogram. Still accidents continued and pilots died even when we found no evidence of heart disease.

Our failure to find evidence of coronary artery disease with the techniques available then had a direct impact on a second problem confronting the Air Force. The Air Force School of Aerospace Medicine was the immediate forerunner of the National Aeronautics and Space Administration (NASA). The scientists and engineers who ultimately would form the nucleus of NASA were beginning to think about reaching the moon, Mars and other planets. It would not look good for a future astronaut to have a heart attack on the moon, or halfway between Earth and Mars. Consequently, among the selection criteria for future astronauts, the absence of heart disease was essential. Since our best medical techniques had failed to detect heart disease in pilots, new and more effective ways to uncover hidden heart disease had to be devised.

So began a lifelong search, not only by myself, but by many cardiologists throughout the world—find better ways to discover heart disease in individuals who appeared to be in good health. My search continued even after I entered clinical practice. Keep in mind that the prevailing way cardiologists practiced their craft in the sixties involved taking a resting blood pressure, listening to the heart with an ordinary stethoscope, an EKG, and a treadmill test—just the way it's done today. If the results of such an examination were negative, and the patient had no symptoms, he was considered to be free from heart disease. Yet, many were the times when a patient was pronounced healthy, only to have a heart attack or die a short time later.

By this time I was in private practice, and the esoteric problems of heart disease in future astronauts was no longer a primary concern. A different kind of challenge faced me. The group of doctors with whom I practiced had a captive patient population of over 35,000 individuals.

They were practicing a new type of health care delivery called pre-paid medicine. In later years it would be called an HMO and become part of the Kaiser organization.

What a splendid source of research material. It didn't take long for me to contact the major pharmaceutical companies and offer our services. Soon we were doing investigational studies on new drugs that had not yet been approved by the FDA. One of these drugs was Edecrin—a product of Merck and Company, one of the largest pharmaceutical companies in the world. Edecrin was a diuretic, but not just another diuretic like the many that had been developed before. No, this behaved differently—it even acted in a different area of the kidney. So powerful was it that one patient with an enormous amount of edema and swelling in her legs and abdomen lost 32 pounds after a single dose!

It is necessary to digress here to explain what edema is, how it can effect the body, and how a diuretic gets rid of edema fluid. The simplest example of edema would be what happens if you cut your hand and it becomes infected. Your hand swells and becomes painful. The swelling is a collection of plasma fluid leaking out of the blood stream into the surrounding tissues. This occurs when blood vessels in the vicinity of the infected area dilate to bring in more white blood cells, the leukocytes. The common name for a large collection of leukocytes is pus. The plasma fluid leaks out of the blood vessels through tiny pores whenever these vessels have to carry a large volume of blood. An increase in volume is accompanied by an increase in pressure. Normally, a certain amount of fluid passes out of the small blood vessels— the capillaries—of the body. An equal amount returns to the capillaries through the process of osmosis. Thus, there is a constant passage of fluid through the vessel's wall as waste products are removed from the tissues. With an infection, more fluid leaks out of the vessel than returns and the delicate balance of osmosis is broken. When the collection of fluid becomes large enough to be seen and felt we call it edema.

Edema may occur for other reasons. For example, in heart failure, the heart is unable to pump a sufficient volume of blood with each heart beat. The blood that is not pumped backs up. This back up of blood reaches all the way to the capillaries, causing an increase in pressure in those tiny vessels. More blood leaks out of the vessels than is pulled back in by osmosis, and the result is edema. Patients with heart failure also secrete a hormone known as aldosterone. This hormone, in turn, stimulates the kidney to retain sodium and water. This is commonly referred to as fluid retention. Since the retained fluid remains within the circulatory system, it eventually causes an increase in pressure and a passage of even more fluid out of the capillaries. Excess aldosterone also is secreted whenever there is emotional stress. If the stress is great enough, fluid retention and edema may take place. The only difference between fluid retention and edema is a matter of degree—if there's enough fluid to be seen it is called edema. Usually there has to be a 10% increase in body weight from fluid retention before it becomes noticeable. Less than this is usually not perceived because the edema fluid distributes itself equally throughout all body tissues. Most patients who are sick enough to retain this much fluid are not very mobile and spend most of their time sitting. At this point gravity will cause the fluid to collect in the legs and ankles. Pressure on the lower leg will cause a deep depression similar to the hole in a mound of clay if you pushed your finger into it.

Diuretics help eliminate edema by acting upon the kidney. Instead of the kidney retaining sodium and water, it allows both to pass right on through to become urine. This is why a diuretic makes you go to the bathroom a lot. The effect of diuretics upon edema can be likened to a sponge filled with water. If the sponge is soaked, even a small amount of squeezing gets rid of a fair amount of water. On the other hand, if the sponge is fairly dry then relatively little water can be squeezed out. Thus, if there is no edema, diuretics may not increase the urine output by much, but they will prevent edema from taking place.

To return now to Edecrin. Why was this such an important drug? Up until the time it was introduced there was no effective diuretic to treat severe heart failure. Conventional diuretics were too weak to eliminate the massive fluid retention we were seeing in our patients. Eventually fluid would accumulate in their lungs—a condition known as pulmonary edema. When this happened their lungs could no longer transfer oxygen to the red blood cells and the victims quickly died of congestive heart failure. Edecrin changed all of that. With a correct dosage the patient would remain edema free and his life would be extended for years.

Those of us who worked with this drug were enormously impressed and gratified. We had always felt so helpless when a patient went into advanced congestive heart failure. Now there was hope at last—we could do something. With the reduction of edema, their shortness of breath and cough would disappear, their heart rate slowed down, their appetite returned, and they no longer had to be confined to bed. They could think, function and be active enough to enjoy life again.

I discussed with the Research Director of Merck and Company the vast improvement in our patients, and told him how good their drug was. I was soberly reminded that most of my observations were subjective, and that they could have resulted from an improvement in the patient's psychological outlook. I was advised that scientific evidence, not subjective feelings by patients, had to be presented to the Food and Drug Administration in order for the drug to be approved. Therefore, I would need objective evidence to prove that the patients were actually better after diuretic therapy.

Once again I had come face to face with the same dilemma— find a group of tests that will detect early heart disease—tests that were far more sensitive than existing ones. If the tests were sensitive enough, we could determine whether a patient had early disease, and whether it was moderate or severe. We would be able to tell when the disease became worse and when it improved. With such tests we could measure the recovery seen after Edecrin administration. Then, and only then, could the subjective improvement be attributed to the new drug.

At about this time, in the mid-sixties, Drs. Alberto Benchimol and E. Gray Dimond were doing their pioneering studies on apexcardiography at the prestigious Scripps Research Institute in La Jolla, California. Around the world other scientists were simultaneously involved in the development of similar procedures—such as the use of systolic time intervals, echocardiography and radioactive imaging—to study heart disease. Within a few years a new field had developed involving the use of all these tests. It was called mechanocardiography—*mechano* meaning mechanical; in other words, having to do with the mechanical function of the heart. This was clearly different from the study of the electrocardiogram, which looked at the electrical output of the heart. The difference between the two were as distinct as the difference between the electrical and motor systems of an automobile. Mechanocardiography soon transformed into the broader field of noninvasive cardiology.

Noninvasive cardiology captured the fancy of many capable cardiologists throughout the world. We had a group of tests that initial studies indicated were highly sensitive for the early detection of heart disease. Moreover, they provided reasonably accurate information about the function of the heart. Soon the new techniques of mechanocardiography, echocardiography and thallium imaging found their way into the evaluation of patients with cardiac disease in many parts of the world.

By this time the restrictions of the HMO I was part of had forced me into solo practice. Fortunately, I was able to take both my patients and equipment with me. Before long I was performing noninvasive procedures routinely on all of my patients. Over the next several years this grew into thousands of recordings and tests on hundreds of patients. In time there was quite a database of patient information including as many as 20 to 30 recordings of cardiac function on many patients.

It soon became apparent that these recordings could be broken down into two separate groups. One consisted of patients whose cardiac function studies were essentially unchanged from year to year, indicating that their disease was stable and had not progressed. The second group of patients had unchanged function studies only up to a point. At that point the studies began to show impaired contraction or relaxation of the heart muscle and abnormal filling of the heart. This suggested that the patient's disease was getting worse. The only problem was that in most of these patients, the abnormalities were unaccompanied by any new symptoms, changes in their physical examination, or EKG changes. This raised the question whether these new tests were providing inaccurate information. Because we didn't have the answer at that time, the observations were temporarily set aside, and the patients were allowed to continue on the same medical program without change.

However, a gnawing doubt began to disturb me—what should I believe, the abnormal cardiac function studies, or the absence of symptoms and the unchanged EKG? The answer to the question was of the utmost importance because the abnormal function studies might be an early warning signal of an impending heart attack. Since most heart attacks occurred without much warning, this could be a major scientific advance.

I could see only one way to solve the problem. Carefully evaluate the patient's clinical status over a period of a year or more, both before and after the changes in cardiac function. Then compare his clinical picture with the clinical picture of patients whose cardiac function was stable. Finally, collect the noninvasive studies in all patients who had died to see if they had anything in common.

The results were striking. In the group with stable cardiac function, as determined by unchanging mechanocardiographic studies, only 3% a year showed some worsening of their cardiac disease as manifested by the appearance of new symptoms, EKG changes, a heart attack or death. In contrast, in those with deteriorating mechanocardiographic function studies, over 80% showed a worsening of their clinical condition in the six months preceding or following the changes. In the 20 patients who had died over a period of several years, a review of their records during the year preceding their death showed that all—100%—had exhibited similar abnormalities!

I noted one other important detail. I had anticipated that any new abnormalities in cardiac function showing up would be from impaired contraction of the heart muscle. This was not an unreasonable assumption since the deprivation of blood flow and oxygen would make it difficult for the heart to contract. While this did occur to some degree, far more common was the impaired relaxation and filling of the heart. This was completely unexpected. Indeed, the changes I noted looked identical to what I saw with fluid overload of the heart in cases of edema. If that were true, then treatment with a diuretic might correct the problem. But fluid retention as a cause of an impending heart attack and unstable angina had never been reported before. Fluid retention occurred in heart failure, but patients with unstable angina were not considered to be in heart failure. How could simple fluid retention in patients not in heart failure *cause* a heart attack?

I began to look more carefully at the information I had. One interesting difference between those patients whose tests remained stable versus those with changing functional studies was their blood pressure. An increased blood pressure as a cause of a heart attack had never been documented, even in our own patients. However, a closer look revealed that while patients with changed heart function still had blood pressures within normal ranges, it was distinctly higher than it had been when their studies were stable. For example, if their resting pressure were 110/65 when stable, it might rise to 140/85 when unstable. Because the latter pressure was still normal, it had escaped notice before these studies. Presumably the rise in blood pressure was a result of the retained fluid entering the circulatory system as a result of edema. This would be like putting air in a tire—the pressure would have

206 / HOW TO PROTECT YOUR HEART

to rise. The rise in blood pressure was sufficient to cause increasing chest pain, the unstable angina, which often preceded a heart attack. This, then, might be the connection between fluid retention, unstable angina and heart attacks.

The next logical step was to administer a diuretic to patients who developed impaired function studies. When such a diuretic was added to the patient's standard medical treatment, in almost every case the mechanocardiographic function studies returned to their prior state. If the diuretic was continued, the patient's clinical course returned to a stable state—no new symptoms. More importantly, the patient's risk of progression of heart disease or its complications was greatly reduced. Keep in mind that none of this information could have been discovered without the sensitive and reliable means of studying the functions of the heart with the new noninvasive procedures.

Now there was a new problem; why did fluid retention occur? This time we had an advantage—it was no longer necessary to go back into past records to reconstruct what was happening. An investigation could be started the same day the deteriorating cardiac function was detected. Soon several possible causes were found. Some patients had a silent urinary tract infection while others had a prostate problem. Both cases lead to an interference with either urine formation or excretion. Clearly this would create some fluid retention. Other patients had been under a considerable amount of recent stress. It was already known that stress could cause fluid retention. Indeed, it was also known that an increase in stress often preceded heart attacks. Perhaps the serial use of mechanocardiographic function studies in patients with coronary artery disease could identify those individuals who did retain fluid with stress. Other causes of fluid retention that could cause changes were weight gain—even small amounts of two to three pounds, excessive food or fluid consumption, and following the use of certain drugs used for pain relief. This latter group of drugs is often referred to as the nonsteroidal, anti-inflammatory drugs or NSAIDS.

You need not be a doctor to predict that if a patient developed impaired cardiac function as a result of a urinary tract infection, then the treatment would not be bypass surgery or angioplasty but an antibiotic to get rid of the infection!

Repeated use of these techniques over a period of years allowed us to make another important observation. The very fact that these tests uncovered deterioration of cardiac function in the complete absence of symptoms was a revelation. It meant that localized myocardial ischemia, a reduction in blood flow to the heart muscle, must be present. Since the myocardial ischemia occurred in the absence of symptoms, it should be more appropriately called silent ischemia.

Doctors had always intuitively assumed that if a cardiac patient had no symptoms, or his existing symptoms were not getting any worse, then his disease was not progressing. Particularly frightening in our modern era, with a high tech solution for every patient with symptoms, is the idea that patients without symptoms were indeed getting worse, even dying. The very existence of silent ischemia challenged that whole fundamental concept of treating only patients with symptoms and eventually led to a major change in the way ischemic heart disease was treated. It was not hard to deduce that if silent ischemia existed, it was not only common but it was progressive. After all, 3,000 individuals had heart attacks every day in the United States alone, and another 1,400 died! In most cases the heart attack occurred without warning. Heart attacks were like earthquakes—the outward manifestations took place without warning, but the underlying forces that went into creating it had been going on for years. The key was silent and progressive myocardial ischemia. Identify it, treat it, and maybe premature heart attacks or sudden death could be prevented!

But how are we to know when silent ischemia is present? The patient doesn't have any symptoms, and the traditional methods of examination are too insensitive to detect it. One way would be with the use of the 24-hour Holter monitor discussed in the last chapter. Indeed, in the late eighties the whole concept of silent ischemia finally received the attention it deserved when advances in the technique of Holter monitoring revealed that silent ischemia was much more common than anyone had ever realized. Moreover, it was found that approximately 75% of ischemic episodes were not accompanied by chest pain.

Another way to detect silent ischemia would be to use serial mechanocardiographic studies over a period of time—apexcardiography, echocardiography, radioactive imaging with thallium, or the use of systolic and diastolic time intervals. Whatever way is used is perfectly acceptable as long as the studies are done in a consistent manner at regular intervals so that the function of the heart can be tracked in an orderly manner.

The inevitable question that must be asked here is should patients without symptoms be treated, and if so, what medications should be used? The following typical case history may provide the answer.

Steve Turner was a 63-year old retired engineer. He had coronary artery disease and had suffered a heart attack eight years previously from which he had a good recovery. He exercised regularly on a treadmill, played golf three times a week, kept his weight down and did not smoke. He hardly ever had angina. Because he was so active and had no symptoms, his doctor felt that medications were not necessary. Three years ago he decided to retire. When he did it was necessary to change health plans and his doctor. He had selected a noninvasive cardiologist whom several of his friends recommended. After an extensive series of tests the cardiologist advised him to begin four different heart medications over the next few months. Initially he worried that his coronary artery disease was getting worse. Why else would the new doctor use so many medications, particularly since his former doctor had said they weren't necessary? The only medication his old doctor said he might need was nitroglycerine underneath his tongue if he ever had any chest pain. His new cardiologist explained that even though he did not have any symptoms, his tests showed that the function of his heart was still significantly impaired from his heart attack. The regular use of the four medications he was recommending would optimize the heart's function. Hopefully, this would have two effects: First, the long range complications of his prior heart attack, such as cardiac enlargement and heart failure, would be retarded or even prevented. Second, if Steve had another heart attack, the medications would cushion the effect and protect him in much the same way that seat belts protected people in an automobile accident. There were other reasons but these were the important ones.

Since the friends who had originally recommended the cardiologist were also taking several medications and were doing well, Steve agreed to cooperate with the recommended medical program. He had some minor side effects to one of the drugs which soon disappeared. On more than one occasion other friends who were going to different cardiologists ridiculed the idea of taking so many "pills." His friend John even opened up his shirt and showed him his bypass surgery scar. "My doctor said I needed immediate surgery when I began having symptoms. Now my coronary circulation is as good as new and I don't need any medication. Maybe your doctor is old fashioned." Another friend, Richard, had his recent symptoms treated with angioplasty and seemed to be doing well with only aspirin. On more than one visit, Steve meant to question his doctor about the variations in treatments. On each occasion, however, the doctor had spent considerable time studying the function of his heart, and had gradually increased his medication with the comment that "things were still not quite perfect." Recently however, no more adjustment in his medication was necessary.

One day Steve was scheduled to play a round of golf with John. When John failed to show up, Steve called his home and was shocked to learn that two days before, he had collapsed at the dinner table and died. Other than the fact that John had been feeling tired for two to three days, his family had no clue that anything was wrong. Two weeks later, his other friend, Richard, had a massive heart attack, went into heart failure and cardiac arrest but was resuscitated. Now his heart needed a pacemaker, and he no longer had the stamina to play golf. Since neither of these two friends had been taking any medication at the time of their catastrophes, Steve decided his cardiologist knew what he was doing.

On a routine visit, his doctor questioned Steve even more closely than usual as to how he felt, whether he was keeping up with his exercise program, was he sure he wasn't having any more chest pain or was he more tired than usual. Steve answered "No" to all the questions but he knew something was wrong. There was. The doctor showed him how his recordings had changed and recommended a small change in his medications. Although he was concerned, the fact that he had no new symptoms made him soon forget the incident. He did agree, however, to take a higher dose of two of his medications.

About one month later, Steve awoke during the night with chest discomfort. It was not severe, certainly not like the pain of his heart attack. He took some nitroglycerine and began to note partial relief; an additional tablet caused the pain to disappear and he went back to sleep. A few hours later he again had chest pain, only this time the pain would not go away. He called his cardiologist. The doctor sent an ambulance and Steve was admitted to the hospital. A short time later he was admitted to the coronary care unit of the same hospital he had been in before. He was not so frightened this time; besides, a shot of morphine on his way through the emergency room had stopped his pain completely. Within minutes the nurse was starting a drip of intravenous nitroglycerine. In the other arm she started an intravenous drip of heparin to prevent his blood from clotting. An electrocardiogram was rapidly done followed by an x-ray in the room. In between all of this a laboratory technician came in and drew some blood for enzyme studies. Shortly thereafter, an echocardiogram was done in his room. He was also given some of the same drugs he was taking at home. By this time the morphine was beginning to have an effect and soon he was asleep.

A few hours later he awoke just as his doctor walked into the room with the electrocardiogram and a computer readout of his enzymes. Steve had had a heart attack, however, it was a mild

211 / *Howard H. Wayne*

one and hopefully, he would have no further symptoms. That, indeed, was exactly what happened. He had only one further episode of chest pain that subsided promptly with nitroglycerine. He learned that his enzymes were only mildly elevated, and the electrocardiogram was already beginning to show improvement. Within two days he was sitting in a chair; in four days he was walking around the room and then the hospital floor, and by seven days he was sent home. Ten days after leaving the hospital he was walking the streets and one month later was back playing golf. His electrocardiogram had returned to its prior state, and he was happily informed that even though he had a heart attack, it left no permanent damage. The medication he had been taking so diligently had finally paid off—a severe or potentially fatal heart attack had been transformed into a minor one with no residual damage. Clearly his doctor had foreseen what was coming and managed to minimize the damage. Steve no longer questioned the need for medication.

The case histories described above are not only true but typical scenarios of what often happens to patients with obstructive coronary artery disease. During the past 15 to 20 years almost all of the heart attack patients I have seen, once they have reached the hospital, have had an exceptionally benign course with rapid recovery, and little in the way of post heart attack disability. I'm referring now to patients who are on a full medical regimen with several different medications, *even though they are not having symptoms*. In contrast, patients on no medical program, or an inadequate one, did not seem to fare too well. Let's take a look at the drugs currently available to see what they do and how they protect the heart.

DRUGS USED TO TREAT OBSTRUCTIVE
CORONARY ARTERY DISEASE

Most of the drugs used to treat ischemic heart disease either reduce the workload of the heart, thereby making it easier for it to contract, or they increase the blood flow to the heart muscle. In some cases a drug will do both. Reducing the workload of the heart is like decreasing one's expenses—there is more money left over at the end of the month. Therefore, if the blood flow through the arteries is restricted, it makes sense to reduce the heart's work so that the amount of blood needed is not greater than what can be delivered.

Increasing the blood flow through the coronary arteries can be likened to increasing one's income. Unfortunately, it may not be possible to accomplish this, or if so, to only a limited degree. First the drugs that reduce the heart's workload.

DRUGS THAT REDUCE THE WORKLOAD OF THE HEART

BETA BLOCKERS

The prototype drug in this class is Inderal. This drug has been available for over 25 years and is still, in my opinion, the most effective of all the beta blockers. Unfortunately, Inderal is often unjustly criticized for too many side effects; consequently, it is frequently ignored in favor of other, less potent beta blockers, and such weaker drugs may result in treatment failure. Inderal combines with chemical receptors on the surface of the heart known as beta-adrenergic receptors. These receptors are chemically structured so that they can combine with certain adrenalin-like hormones secreted by the body. These hormones are naturally discharged whenever the heart has to increase its rate, or its force of contraction. Thus, whenever your heart rate goes from 70 to 100, and you feel it pumping in your chest, it's because of these adrenaline-like substances. One is called adrenaline, the other noradrenaline. It matters not what the stimulus is—playing tennis or having a fight with your boss—when these substances are secreted, your heart rate and blood pressure increase. This will quickly produce chest pain in individuals with obstructive coronary artery disease.

Beta blockers act by combining with the chemical receptors on the heart's surface to prevent the increase in heart rate caused by adrenaline and noradrenaline. Therefore, with beta blockers the heart does not require as much oxygen or blood flow as it did before, and chest pain is prevented.

Beta blockers are also highly effective in the long term treatment of high blood pressure, which also increases the workload of the heart. Many individuals with hypertension will experience an increase in heart rate, blood pressure and the force of the heart's contraction with any increase in stress. Inderal prevents this from happening.

The usual dose of Inderal is about 160 mg per day. Occasionally, a patient will require twice that amount. Conversely, some patients require as little as 40 mg per day. How do we determine how much to give? Simply by timing the heart rate. An effective dose usually brings the heart rate down to about 50-60 per minute. Any rate lower than 50 may mean the patient is taking too much. Decisions about dosage have to be individualized because some people have a natural heart rate of 60. In such cases, a less than effective dose may bring the heart rate down to 55 per minute. Accordingly, other criteria have to be used.

While there is little danger of someone with a vigorously contracting heart receiving too much Inderal in the standard doses, a patient with a poorly contracting heart may have profound side effects to beta blockers. Such a person may be in mild heart failure from several prior heart attacks. As a result, his heart may be so badly damaged and enlarged that it has lost its elasticity, and is too weak to contract effectively. When the heart is unable to pump enough blood with each heart beat, it will speed up so there are more beats per minute. In this way the total output of the heart per minute fulfills the needs of the body. This is one of our compensatory mechanisms. In these subjects, the administration of as little as 40 mg of Inderal might slow the heart rate so much that profound weakness occurs. Fortunately, this does not happen very often. Inderal remains an outstandingly effective drug in the vast majority of patients in whom it is used properly.

Even in the absence of angina or hypertension, beta blockers have been shown to protect against future heart attacks and to reduce mortality after a heart attack, when given on a chronic basis. Studies also show a reduction in mortality when beta blockers are used during an acute heart attack. One precaution should be emphasized, however. Beta blockers must never be stopped abruptly. To do so may cause the very heart attack you are trying to avoid. It is all right to discontinue such drugs gradually over a period of one to two weeks.

The various beta blocker drugs in common usage beside Inderal include Tenormin, Lopressor, Normodyne, and Corgard. Most doctors tend to use one or two of these in their daily practice. If a given beta blocker causes a side effect, then switching to a different agent may eliminate that problem. While the list of side effects reported with these drugs is very long, I have seen relatively few in actual practice with appropriate doses. These include hair loss, a decrease in exercise tolerance, insomnia, a decreased ability to concentrate, impotence and cold hands or feet. The actual percentage of patients who have one or more of the above side effects is probably less than 10%.

CALCIUM CHANNEL BLOCKERS

The calcium channel blockers are an entirely different class of drugs. These drugs act by relaxing the muscular walls of all arteries in the body including the coronary vessels. Relaxation of the musculature of a coronary artery will increase its diameter and enable it to carry more blood and oxygen to the heart muscle. In addition, since all other arteries throughout the body are affected, there will be a decrease in the resistance to the flow of blood, and a fall in blood pressure. The final effect will be a reduction in the work the heart must do, and a decrease in its need for oxygen.

The most commonly used of the calcium channel blockers is Cardizem. A number of others are in widespread use and include Procardia, Calan (also known as Isoptin), Cardene, DynaCirc, Norvasc and Vascor. The advantage of these calcium channel blockers is their dual effect of lowering blood pressure while increasing coronary blood flow.

Precautions are needed because some of the calcium channel blockers will slow the heart rate if given to patients who are already taking beta blockers. These same drugs can depress the function of the heart and precipitate heart failure, particularly in patients who already have depressed cardiac function. The drugs most likely to cause this are Procardia, Calan or Isoptin, and Cardizem. There are other minor side effects associated with these drugs, too, but their frequency is small and they are not clinically significant. In general, the calcium channel blocking agents are highly effective, safe, and when used with care, can be depended upon to provide considerable benefit in most patients with angina and hypertension.

ACE INHIBITORS

Angiotensin converting enzyme inhibitors, more popularly referred to as the ACE inhibitors are often used in angina and post heart attack patients. Angiotensin is a hormone produced by the body that elevates blood pressure. In order for this hormone to work, a converting enzyme is necessary to change its structure. ACE inhibitors prevent this chemical change from happening. Strictly speaking these are not anti-anginal drugs. However, they are highly effective in lowering the blood pressure. Remember, a normal blood pressure is too high for someone with heart disease. Experience has shown that the patient with a low blood pressure has less chest pain and fewer heart attacks. Accordingly, pressure should be reduced to the lowest level possible, as long as it doesn't interfere with the patient's activities. I have found that adding ACE inhibitors to an existing medical program, usually lowers blood pressure without side effects. Without ACE inhibitors other drugs aren't as effective, except in very high doses.

In addition to lowering blood pressure, ACE inhibitors inhibit the changes that take place after a heart attack that lead to the heart's enlargement and loss of its elasticity. The prototype ACE inhibitor is Capoten. Vasotec is another useful drug. Unfortunately, both these medications have to be taken twice a day. Newer ACE inhibitors such as Zestril or Prinivil, Lotensin, Altace and Monopril only have to be taken once a day and are extremely effective.

DRUGS THAT INCREASE CORONARY BLOOD FLOW

NITROGLYCERINE AND NITRATES

Nitroglycerine and nitrates have been used to treat patients with chest pain due to coronary artery disease for over 100 years. In the early part of this century, doctors noticed that munitions workers processing nitroglycerine for explosives would develop chest pain on weekends. However, their symptoms would be relieved when they returned to work on Mondays. It was found they were absorbing nitroglycerine through their lungs and skin from the fumes surrounding them. By Fridays, they had a high concentration of the drug in their body tissues, but over the weekend the level of nitroglycerine gradually decreased and the angina would return.

Two kinds of nitroglycerine drugs are available. One is the sublingual tablet that is placed beneath the tongue, is promptly absorbed, and affects the coronary blood flow within two to three minutes. It is actually called a nitroglycerine tablet and goes by the trade name of Nitrostat. Nitroglycerine also is manufactured as an oral spray, as an ointment and in patches that can be applied to the skin where it is absorbed into the blood stream in 20 to 30 minutes.

The second type of nitroglycerine preparation manufactured is a compound known as nitrates. This comes as an oral tablet or as a special tablet that can be placed beneath the tongue. When placed beneath the tongue, effects begin within five minutes, while the effects of the oral tablets do not start until 30-45 minutes. The sublingual tablets only last about 30 minutes while the oral tablet lasts for 6-8 hours.

Nitrates take longer to be metabolized than nitroglycerine. Both nitroglycerine and nitrates produce a substance that is normally secreted by the cells lining the walls of the coronary arteries. That substance is known as nitric oxide. It has a powerful relaxing effect on the muscle cells within the arterial wall allowing the artery to dilate and carry more blood. The most commonly used form of nitrate is Isordil. Its generic name is isosorbide dinitrate.

Nitroglycerine and nitrates not only dilate the coronary arteries, they preferentially dilate the small veins throughout the body known as venules. Venules are the smallest veins in the circulatory system through which blood flows immediately after it leaves the capillaries. There are a tremendous number of such venules in the body, and they are capable of storing a considerable amount of blood. Consequently, after nitroglycerine is given, there is an increase in the blood carrying capacity on the venous side of the circulation. The result is a reduction in the amount of blood returning to the heart, a decrease in the volume of blood within the heart's chambers with each heart beat, and a fall in pressure within the heart's chambers. Accordingly, there is less compression of the microcirculation and an increase in coronary blood flow.

Nitroglycerine and nitrates are extremely effective in relieving chest pain, as well as some of the other symptoms of coronary artery disease. Unfortunately, their efficacy has been greatly limited by a lack of understanding of a phenomena known as nitroglycerine tolerance. We now know that patients can develop a tolerance to the circulatory effects of nitroglycerine and nitrates within a few days of first taking the drug. Consequently, the ability of these drugs to dilate blood vessels, and their effectiveness in relieving chest pain is rapidly lost.

Up until the early eighties, it was believed that nitroglycerine and nitrates lost their ability to relieve angina because of their rapid disappearance from the circulation. The pharmaceutical industry found an answer for this: they developed a unique type of patch that allowed continuous absorption of nitroglycerine through the skin. It became possible to maintain a therapeutic level in the blood stream for 24 hours per patch.

The nitroglycerine patch was a triumph of technology. Unfortunately it failed to relieve the problem. Patients still obtained relief for a few days to a week, but then the benefits were lost, even though the blood concentration of nitroglycerine was still high. Clearly, their arteries and veins had lost their ability to respond and had become tolerant of the drug. It was soon realized that the only way this tolerance could be removed was by giving patients a nitroglycerine free interval of about 12 hours each day. Today, nitroglycerine and nitrates are so successful that when used in conjunction with other anti-anginal agents, and in proper doses, most patients are able to achieve complete relief of their symptoms.

Despite the efficacy of nitroglycerine and nitrates, doctors frequently fail to prescribe an adequate dosage. Using Isordil, the most widely prescribed nitrate as an example, the maximal dosage prescribed is often no more than 10-20 milligrams three times a day. In my experience, 40-80 milligrams, two to three times a day, is often required for the desired effect. Isordil is perfectly safe to take, and headaches are its most annoying side effect. These generally subside after the first week or two. If not, Tylenol or aspirin may be taken along with the nitrate until the headaches subside spontaneously. It is wise to have an interval of at least 12 hours between the evening and morning doses to avoid developing tolerance.

The most popular nitrates besides Isordil are Sorbitrate, Cardilate, Dilatrate, and Peritrate. It may be necessary to give each of these in multiples of two to four times the recommended starting dose to gain relief from symptoms. Nitroglycerine skin patches include Minitran, Nitro-Dur and Transderm-Nitro. Nitroglycerine also can be administered as an ointment. It is somewhat messy and more inconvenient than the patches; nevertheless, it is just as effective and considerably less expensive. Commonly used ointments include Nitrol, and Nitrostat.

Aside from headaches, the most frequently encountered side effects derive from the ability of these drugs to dilate blood vessels throughout the body. The most important of these reactions is a fall in blood pressure. When this happens the subject is apt to experience weakness, dizziness and a faint feeling, particularly when standing upright. In rare instances fainting may occur, especially when nitrates are used in association with other drugs such as beta blockers, calcium channel blockers and diuretics. In the majority of such cases, the patient will have taken all these medications on an empty stomach and delayed having a meal.

The result is a too rapid absorption of the medications into the blood stream with a fall in blood pressure. These side effects can be controlled by a reduction in dosage, or by taking the medication after meals.

DIURETICS

Most doctors use only beta blockers, calcium channel blockers and nitrates in the treatment of angina pectoris. Few seem to be aware that one of the most effective drugs for this condition is diuretics. You will recall from earlier in this chapter that fluid retention occurs when there is abnormal retention of sodium and water by the kidneys, and that it may occur for several different reasons. Such fluid retention is extremely common, but most victims are totally unaware it is present. The signs are recognizable by those familiar with it and include mild puffiness under the eyes, some difficulty in removing rings from the fingers, a feeling that shoes are tight, particularly after sitting for prolonged periods, and a tightness of snug fitting clothes. The tightness also reflects the increase in pressure within the tissues. Women tend to be more familiar with this feeling than men because they experience premenstrual fluid retention. The female breast tends to be fuller and more tender in such circumstances. Typically these are subjective feelings experienced by the patient and not objective signs that a doctor will notice. Not until there is a great deal of fluid retention will a doctor note its presence, and by this time it is severe enough to be called edema.

I have already mentioned when I first began to use mechanocardiographic studies on a routine basis in patients with coronary artery disease, I serendipitously found that some patients developed abnormal heart function that appeared to be due to fluid retention. This fluid retention may have been due to the very drugs I was using to treat the disease. For reasons we don't entirely understand, fluid retention is seen following the use of beta blockers, nitrates and some calcium channel blockers. This can have a profound influence on the effectiveness of nitrates because this fluid is distributed equally throughout the body tissues where it can cause an increase in tissue pressure. Nitrates act, in part, by dilating the venules of the body. Venules have no protection as do the arteries. There are no muscular fibers within their walls to resist compression or collapse. Consequently, they are quite susceptible to such compression whenever fluid retention causes the tissues of the body to swell and the tissue pressure to increase. If enough venules are compressed, the reservoir function of these vessels is eliminated. Therefore, whenever there is fluid retention, the effectiveness of nitrates is lost. Indeed, this may be one of the mechanisms to account for the development of tolerance to these drugs.

Diuretics can prevent all this from happening. Usually it is necessary to take them both morning and evening. When this is done, regardless of the cause of the fluid retention, diuretics will eliminate the excess fluid from the body. On occasion, the standard diuretic drugs such as HydroDiuril (hydrochlorothiazide) will not work, particularly if kidney disease is present. In this situation the stronger loop diuretics such as Lasix or Edecrin are necessary. Because diuretics also help to lower the blood pressure, these drugs, when used with other anti-anginal medications, are extremely effective in relieving symptoms.

Many doctors seem to be reluctant to use diuretics under the false premise that they cause side effects that are harmful. The most important side effect is a loss of potassium accompanying the excretion of sodium and water from the body. This danger is greatly exaggerated. When standard doses of diuretics are used, significant potassium loss is not likely to occur, particularly if the patient is taking supplementary potassium or a potassium blocking agent. Nonetheless, the occurrence of low potassium, hypokalemia, may occur in some patients, and it can be serious.

There are three ways to avoid the development of hypokalemia. One way is to simply eat more potassium rich foods such as bananas. This is often difficult to do, and may increase the caloric intake significantly. For example, it has been estimated that it is necessary to eat approximately five feet of bananas a day to avoid potassium loss. Unless you happen to be an ape, it might be hard to stomach such a diet. A second way to maintain the blood level of potassium is to take potassium pills. These are certainly more palatable and are widely used. The problem with this approach is that the greater the potassium intake, the more potassium is excreted in the urine. This is like running in place—a lot of effort is expended but you don't get anyplace. The third way to prevent potassium loss is to take a potassium blocking agent along with the diuretic. These drugs work by preventing potassium loss through the kidney. They are highly effective and very safe. Three such drugs are in common use—Midamor, Dyrenium and Aldactone.

Other side effects of diuretics have been overemphasized to a degree that is ridiculous. These include transient elevations of blood sugar, cholesterol and uric acid. The cholesterol elevation effect is the one that has created the greatest amount of misunderstanding. Some worry that since diuretics elevate the cholesterol level, the patient is at an increased risk of having a heart attack. This is nothing but gross distortion of the facts. Indeed, not taking the diuretic is far more likely to cause a heart attack. Yes, cholesterol level is mildly increased by diuretics, but the degree of increase is so small as to make such claims ludicrous. Furthermore, any increase is only transient—within a few months the body adjusts and returns to its prior level. Similarly, patients have mild elevations of the blood sugar and uric acid levels, but the increase is not enough to be clinically significant, considering the overwhelming benefit of diuretic therapy. Moreover, any increase in levels can be neutralized by medications designed to lower them, if it is really necessary.

Commonly used standard diuretics known as the thiazide diuretics include HydroDiuril, Diuril, Esidrex, Enduron, Hydromox, Lozol, Oretic and Zaroxolyn. Standard diuretics may be combined with a potassium retaining diuretic and can be obtained as Moduretic, Maxide, Dyazide and Aldactazide. The more potent loop diuretics include Lasix, Edecrin, Bumex and Demadex.

ASPIRIN

Aspirin is different from the drugs discussed thus far in that it has no direct effect upon the heart. It is an anti-platelet drug. Platelets are cellular constituents of the blood in the same way as red and white blood cells. When subjected to trauma, they liberate a substance that aids in the formation of a clot. As blood passes over an irregular arteriosclerotic plaque in the wall of a coronary artery, it is not unlike driving over a bump or ditch in the road— the car receives a jolt. So does the blood. Platelets are traumatized and small amounts of clot-like material are laid down. Sometimes a large clot may form and cause an acute occlusion. Aspirin interrupts this sequence. Studies on many thousands of patients with chronic heart disease have shown that one-half an aspirin a day will result in about a 10% reduction in mortality and about a 30% decrease in the occurrence of nonfatal heart attacks. When taken at the onset of an acute heart attack, there is a similar benefit. Aspirin helps in the prevention of the complications of heart disease, and I suggest that all my patients use it.

SHOULD PATIENTS WITH SILENT ISCHEMIA BE TREATED?

To return now to the question posed earlier in this chapter— should patients with chronic ischemia, but without symptoms be treated, and if so, what medications should be used?

Many patients with coronary artery disease have chronic ischemia, and most ischemia is silent. While the majority do not have chest pain, many suffer from fatigue as their limiting symptom. This leads most patients to avoid those activities that tire them. Both patient and doctor are deceived into believing that symptoms are absent. Inevitably this inactivity engenders a certain amount of deconditioning that leads to further exertional fatigue and further deconditioning. This cycle will have a negative impact on cardiovascular function. It should come as no surprise that in these individuals, silent ischemia has the same ominous prognosis as symptomatic ischemia, and results in progressive deterioration of cardiac function. Therefore, the first reason that silent myocardial ischemia should be treated is to prevent the vicious circle of deconditioning.

The second reason why silent ischemia should be treated is to prevent its complications. Whenever there is damage to an area of heart muscle, and it is unable to move, the segment on the opposite wall will compensate by contracting more forcefully. In this way the same amount of compression of the heart's chamber takes place, but one wall of the heart may have to move twice the distance as it once did. In time this causes the harder working segment to stretch and the heart enlarges. Whenever this happens, the work of the heart increases, stimulating further stretching and enlargement. Eventually, the muscle loses its elasticity and the heart begins to fail. Once heart failure begins, about 50% of patients will die within just a few years. It would seem logical that prevention of ischemia would prevent this cascade of events from taking place.

The third reason for medical treatment is to protect the patient by either preventing or minimizing a heart attack. The case history presented earlier in this chapter is an example of such protection.

As a rule, evidence of ischemia can be demonstrated with one or more noninvasive tests recorded either at rest or during stress. If this ischemia can be decreased or eliminated with any of the medications mentioned in this chapter, then that patient should be maintained on those drugs as long as the ischemia exists. My own practice is to begin with beta blockers and diuretics. If necessary, I will add a nitrate preparation in increasing dosages until I obtain the desired effect or until side effects such as headaches, limits the dosage. If hypertension is present, I will add an ACE inhibitor in an attempt to reduce the blood pressure to the lowest possible value. As a rule, one aspirin every other day is also added.

What is the outcome of such a medical program. In my own practice where serial mechanocardiographic and other noninvasive tests are used regularly to optimize treatment, heart attacks are extremely rare—less than one percent a year. Similarly, unexpected or premature death is even more rare—probably no more than 0.5% a year. Only two of my patients have been sent for bypass surgery in the past 12 years and only three had angioplasty. Thus, more heroic forms of treatment clearly have been avoided in almost every case. These values are far less than the heart attack rate and mortality that follows treatment with bypass surgery or angioplasty.

A good medical program will allow a patient to be symptom free and enjoy a normal life span in most cases. Whether this happens or not depends entirely upon the ability of the cardiologist to identify patients with silent ischemia who stand to benefit the most from a medical program similar to the one described in this chapter. Patients with symptoms will always be treated for they demand attention. It is those without symptoms who have the most to gain, and the most to lose if they are ignored. If you have coronary artery disease, your survival will largely depend upon who treats you and the course of therapy he chooses. So choose your doctor well!

AFTERWORD

A sacred trust of the heart

ONCE UPON A TIME doctors had a sacred trust, not only with their patients but with other doctors as well. As we approach the end of this century, it seems that trust is also coming to an end. In part this is because the responsibility for patient care has shifted from the single doctor and patient to the divided care of groups of specialists taking care of groups of patients. Also, the doctor-patient relationship has been significantly influenced by such outside forces as the federal government, hospitals, insurance companies, managed health care plans, employers, the pharmaceutical industry, medical equipment manufacturers and other members of the health care industry. Collectively these forces have been called the medical-industrial complex. [1]

Many people feel the medical-industrial complex caters to overzealous and overtrained specialists, and encourages them to overutilize expensive equipment and overtreat patients with relatively benign diseases. Their purpose is to fill the operating rooms, subsidize the diagnostic laboratories, keep the surgeons, nurses, technicians and other support people busy, and fill the empty beds. This is an important reason why medicine has become technology driven and profit oriented. It also explains why so many patients receive expensive tests and costly treatments that are not needed. Paradoxically, it is frequently not known whether a new technology is more effective, or even more cost beneficial than that which it replaced. Moreover, new technology often doesn't replace older technology, but is merely added on to it.

This overuse of technology is the major reason for the high cost of medical care. Because of that overuse and high cost, a revolution in health care delivery has taken place, ostensibly to lower health care costs. In reality, the managed health care plans that have evolved recently to accomplish this are themselves integral players in the medical-industrial complex. In other words, their real purpose it to capitalize on the enormous profits that can be made by making it appear that health care is being delivered at a lower cost. As we have seen, costs are not lowered, they are merely shifted to non-managed care patients. Furthermore, managed care often leads to a choice between quality of medical care and the saving of lives. When that choice runs head on against the profit motive, then a decision is usually made favoring profit, even if it means poorer quality medical care and loss of patient lives.

The doctor is as much a victim of this situation as is his patient. The profession he loves is being ravished by outside forces that emphasize cost control and profits rather than the needs and welfare of patients, and he is helpless to stop them. On one hand he sees patients whose health or life may be destroyed from denial of essential health care services. At the opposite extreme, the same effect may occur from the overuse and abuse of technology. Worst of all, because he is unable to properly inform his patients as to what is happening, he finds himself unable to maintain the sacred trust that he once had with every patient. Dr. Arnold Relman, the former editor of the New England Journal of Medicine defines trust as follows: "the physician is obligated to act as the trustee for the patient's interest, and whenever possible, with the patient's informed consent. The patient's interest takes precedence over all other considerations —certainly over any financial or other personal interests of the physician."[2]

Nowadays, we even see a loss of trust between the physicians who do research and those who apply the results to patients. Commonly the funding for such research is from a member of the medical-industrial-complex. Inevitably, this introduces a considerable amount of bias and conflict of interest. Accordingly, and for self-serving reasons, medical researchers increasingly make exaggerated claims in published articles as to the effectiveness of new treatments, and minimize their side effects and the unpredictability of the results. In reality, such articles are nothing more than medical advertisements. Medical journals are filled with such trash. An article might state that treatment A is highly effective in selected patients with heart disease with a relatively low risk of side effects. The article does not state that the number benefited is small, that there is no way to predict in advance who will be benefited and who will be made worse, that the side effects will be considerably greater with less skilled doctors, and that treatment is very expensive. Nevertheless, a newspaper might eagerly report such an item with headlines describing the "new treatment." A trusting physician may recommend such a treatment only to have his patient develop unexpected complications from what is really an experimental procedure. Sadly, neither the doctor nor his patient recognize that both they and the news media have been exploited. The result is a misinformation explosion that leads directly to mistreatment. The only ones who profit from such abuses are the medical researchers and the medical-industrial-complex who sell their products.

Yet, there is hope. The practice of medicine, as we know it, is being bombarded from all sides by new technology and treatments, rising costs and new forms of health care delivery. The confluence of these forces is reshaping the future of medical care and how doctors practice medicine. It is up to the public to accept or reject whatever emerges, for it will be our heritage to pass on. Underdiagnosis and undertreatment, overdiagnosis and overtreatment, and medical experimentation rather than established medical treatment can only take place when the patient is uninformed. By taking responsibility for your own health care needs, and thinking of yourself as an informed consumer, both you and your doctor can avoid becoming victims of what is happening. Moreover, your informed interest will help guide how medicine is practiced in the future. I hope this book will help us all reach that goal.

REFERENCES

1.Relman, A.S. The new medical-industrial complex. *N Eng J Med*, 1980; 303: 963-70.

2.Relman, A.S. Shattuck Lecture. The health care industry: Where is it taking us? *N Eng J Med*, 1991; 325: 854-59.

GLOSSARY

ACE inhibitor: A class of drug that lowers blood pressure by blocking the action of a blood pressure hormone known as Angiotensin II.

Angina Pectoris or Angina: Chest pain due to temporary reduction in blood flow to the heart muscle. It has a unique feeling and is often described as if someone were sitting on the patient's chest, or as a constricting band around the chest.

Angiogenesis: The development of new blood vessels that grow out upstream from an obstructed artery and connect to a healthy artery so that blood can flow around the obstruction.

Aorta: The main artery exiting from the heart.

Beta Blocker: A class of drugs that slows the heart rate and reduces the work load of the heart by blocking the actions of adrenalin-like hormones.

Calcium Channel Blocker: A class of drug that both lowers blood pressure and increases the flow of blood in the coronary arteries.

Catheterization: The placement of plastic tubes called catheters within the heart's chambers in order to visualize the inside of the heart and its valves as well as measure the pressures within the chambers and the output of the heart.

Cerebral ischemia: Reduced blood flow to the brain.

Collateral vessels: When a coronary artery is obstructed new blood vessels will bud out from the artery upstream from the obstruction and reinsert into the mother artery downstream from the obstruction. Alternatively, blood vessels will arise from a nearby healthy artery and connect with an obstructed vessel downstream from the blockage. In either case blood flow will be maintained. These new vessels are called collateral vessels.

Coronary Angiogram: This is a procedure in which a flexible catheter (a long plastic tube) is inserted into a femoral artery (the main artery in the upper thigh). The catheter is pushed up into the femoral artery until it reaches the aorta (the main artery in the chest and abdomen). The cardiologist continues to push the catheter up the aorta until it reaches the heart. At this point the catheter is manipulated until it enters one of the main coronary arteries on the surface of the heart. When it is firmly within the coronary artery, a dye solution is injected under pressure so that it can fill the entire arterial tree. The dye is opaque to x-rays; consequently, when an x-ray is taken, the coronary artery and all its branches are seen. If the artery is narrowed, it is assumed it is due to coronary artery disease caused by arteriosclerosis.

Coronary Arteries: The arteries on the surface of the heart that supply blood to the muscle. They arise from the aorta as soon as it exits from the heart.

Coronary Angioplasty: A procedure in which a special catheter with an inflatable balloon at the end is introduced into a coronary artery and guided to the area where the artery is maximally narrowed. Here the balloon is inflated with pressures ranging from 32 to more than 200 pounds per square inch (it takes about 32 pounds per square inch to inflate an automobile tire). The goal is to compress or disrupt the arteriosclerotic plaque so that the vessel becomes less narrowed.

Coronary Artery Bypass Surgery: The insertion of a new vessel into a coronary artery before and after an obstruction so that blood can bypass the narrowed area. Typically, one end of the new vessel is inserted into the aorta immediately after it exits from the heart. The other end is inserted into the obstructed artery beyond the point of obstruction.

Coronary Artery Disease: Arteriosclerosis of the coronary arteries on the surface of the heart (hardening of the arteries).

Coronary Artery Dissection: A complication of angioplasty. When an artery is stretched, the inside lining of the artery may tear. Blood enters the wall of the artery and causes its muscular layers to separate. As a result, the artery may rupture, or the lumen of the artery may collapse and block the passage of blood causing a heart attack.

Coronary artery restenosis: When a section of a coronary artery that was treated with balloon angioplasty becomes narrowed or obstructed again.

Diastolic Pressure: The bottom number of the blood pressure reading. It reflects the pressure within the arteries while the heart is relaxing. A diastolic pressure greater than 85 is abnormal.

Diuretic: A drug that will increase the flow of urine and eliminate excess fluid retained by the body.

Echocardiogram: Sonar imaging of the inside of the beating heart taken from the surface of the chest. It allows the viewer to see the contraction and relaxation of the heart muscle, the opening and closing of the four heart valves, the chambers of the heart and its geometry. Accurate measurements can be obtained of the thickness of the heart muscle and the dimensions of the cardiac chambers.

Edema: Fluid in the tissues creating a swelling.

Electrocardiogram (EKG): A recording of the electrical output of the heart. Electrodes are attached to all four extremities and also placed at various locations on the surface of the chest in the vicinity of the heart.   The recording reflects the electrical activity generated by the heart during its contraction and relaxation.

Health Care Industry: Companies and entities involved in the diagnosis and treatment of patients, the delivery of such care and its payment. It includes doctors, nurses, paramedical people, medical schools, hospitals, insurance companies, pharmaceutical companies, manufacturers of equipment for the diagnosis and treatment of disease and anyone involved in medical care.

Heart attack: This is the lay term used to describe sudden and complete blockage of a major coronary artery. The heart muscle nourished by that artery either will be injured or will die depending upon the amount of residual blood flow to the area. The medical term for heart attack is myocardial infarction.

Heart failure: Failure of the heart to supply the body with the necessary blood to survive. Usually it is due to damage to the heart muscle caused by lack of blood from coronary artery disease or infection. It also may be caused by high blood pressure or damage to the heart valves so that the heart becomes extremely enlarged, stretched and loses its elasticity. Ultimately, the heart muscle becomes too weak to pump blood to the body.

HMO or Health Maintenance Organization: An HMO is one form of a managed health care plan. It differs from the usual managed health care plan in that the HMO provides both the financing of health care, and the providing of it by hiring the doctors. In return for this service, the patient pays a fixed monthly fee. HMO doctors are restricted by the HMO guidelines on the diagnostic tests they are allowed to use and how patients should be treated. HMO doctors can only service members who belong to the HMO.

Hypertension: The medical term for high blood pressure.

Hypertensive angina: Chest pain similar to ordinary angina but lasting longer and due to acute elevations of the blood pressure.

Hypokalemia: A low potassium level in the blood usually caused by excess diuretics in conjunction with reduced food intake, fever or diarrhea.

Ischemia: Reduced blood flow to a tissue, organ or area of the body.

Isometric hand grip stress: A simple stress test accomplished by maximally squeezing a spring-loaded grip device for about one minute. It can cause an acute and significant increase in blood pressure, heart rate and work load upon the heart.

Lumen: The inside of an artery.

Managed Health Care Plan: Managed health plans only provide for the financing of health care. They may contract with doctors to provide health care at a predetermined discounted fee, but they do not hire them. The doctor, in turn, agrees to provide care at this fee. Like the HMO doctors, physicians who contract with managed health care plans also are restricted in the diagnostic tests they are allowed to use and how patients should be treated. Unlike HMO doctors, physicians who contract with managed care plans can service patients from several different plans.

Mechanocardiography: A group of noninvasive tests that record the mechanical function of the heart, in contrast to the electrocardiogram which only records the electrical output of the heart.

Myocardial Infarction: See under *Heart attack* above.

Myocardial ischemia: Reduced blood flow to the heart muscle.

Myocardium: Heart muscle.

Nitroglycerine tablets: A drug that when placed beneath the tongue will cause an increase in blood flow to the heart muscle in two to three minutes by enlarging the coronary arteries and lowering the blood pressure.

Noninvasive: The term used for tests that do not require penetration of the skin or the placement of tubes within the body.

Placebo: A pill containing only sugar. It is often used in scientific experiments in order to make a test subject think he is receiving a medication. If improvement in symptoms occur on placebo medications, the improvement can be attributed to spontaneous healing or to a psychological effect.

Platelets: Cellular components of the blood that help in the clotting of blood.

Systolic Pressure: The top number of a blood pressure reading. It refers to the pressure within the heart's chambers and within the arteries when the heart is contracting and blood is entering the circulation. A systolic pressure above 140 is considered abnormal.

Ventricular Fibrillation: Sudden failure of the heart to contract. Muscle contraction is replaced by tiny rippling movements. Unless fibrillation is terminated and muscle contraction restored within four minutes, brain death will occur.

INDEX